STEPHAN BEUER
MARTIN STANGL
EDWARD P. ALLEN

BASIC DENTAL SUTURING
A PRACTICAL HANDBOOK

Stephan Beuer
Martin Stangl
Edward P. Allen

Basic Dental Suturing

A Practical Handbook

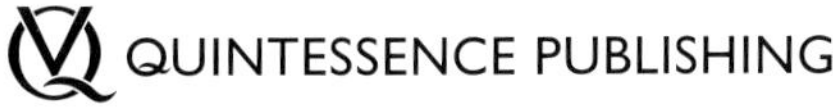

Berlin | Chicago | Tokyo
Barcelona | London | Milan | Mexico City | Paris | Prague | Seoul | Warsaw
Beijing | Istanbul | Sao Paulo | Zagreb

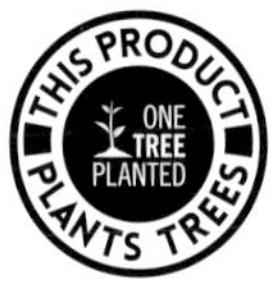

One book, one tree: In support of reforestation worldwide and to address the climate crisis, for every book sold Quintessence Publishing will plant a tree (https://onetreeplanted.org/).

Numerous videos are included in this book that illustrate the content and enrich the reading experience. These can easily be played via QR code using a smartphone or tablet.

Alternatively, the videos can also be accessed via this link:
https://video.qvnet.de/b24331/

Title of original issue:
Der rote Faden
Dentalchirurgische Nahttechniken

A CIP record for this book is available from the British Library.
ISBN: 978-1-78698-123-3

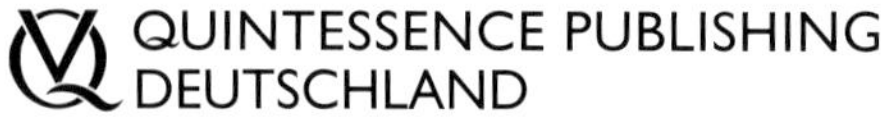

Quintessenz Verlags-GmbH
Ifenpfad 2–4
12107 Berlin
Germany
www.quintessence-publishing.com

Quintessence Publishing Co Ltd
Grafton Road, New Malden
Surrey KT3 3AB
United Kingdom
www.quintessence-publishing.com

Editing: Quintessence Publishing Co, Inc, Batavia, IL, USA
Layout, Production and Reproduction: Quintessenz Verlags-GmbH, Berlin, Germany

Printed and bound in Croatia by Grafički zavod Hrvatske d.o.o.

For Josephina and Korbinian, Felix, and Tim

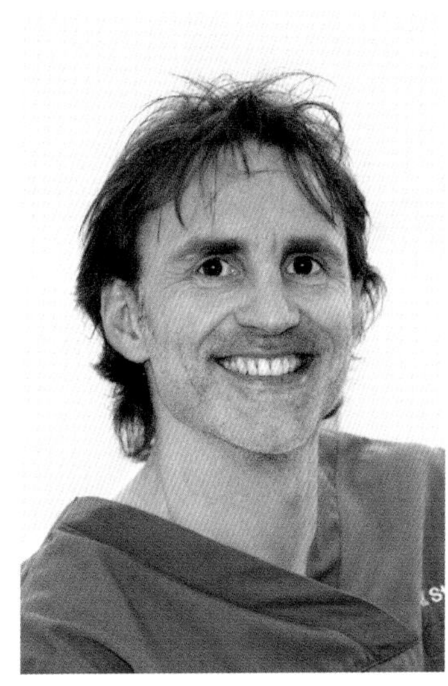

Foreword

Implantology and periodontal plastic surgery have become an integral part of reconstructive dentistry. The purely functional indication of implantology for the replacement of natural tooth roots, for static abutment augmentation, or for fixed tooth restoration has long since changed to esthetic implant reconstruction. In addition to the imitation of white tooth structure, the reconstruction of lost hard and soft tissue is a basic prerequisite for this. The techniques for hard and soft tissue augmentation in particular are very technique sensitive and require a great deal of practice and skill on the part of the surgeon. Especially in hard tissue augmentation, primary wound closure and primary wound healing are of extreme importance because any wound dehiscence will lead to postoperative problems, resulting in complications or failure. Gentle and atraumatic intraoperative treatment of the soft tissues is crucial for irritation-free primary wound healing. The correct incision and flap design with well-perfused flaps, the precise preparation of the flaps at different thicknesses, and tension-free wound closure are all important. Correct suturing techniques are required to ensure this. Suture materials and needle selection also play an important role here. Appropriate wound closure thus contributes massively to the success of the surgical procedure and also represents a high proportion of the time required for the procedure. The saying "many sutures are the death of wounds" dates back to times when relatively thick needle-thread combinations were used to close wounds. With the advent of microsurgery in periodontal plastic surgery and subsequently in implantology, we can now fix and adapt the wound margins very carefully and securely with thin needle-suture combinations in a relatively atraumatic manner.

Unfortunately, the topic of suturing is given far too little attention in many textbooks, and little is said about safe wound closure, especially in the area of hard tissue augmentation. I am therefore particularly pleased that these two authors have addressed this very important topic in this book and presented it so clearly. This book can be regarded as a supplement to all implantology and periodontology books.

In addition, this text is intended to give students and young professionals a good overview of the various suture techniques that can be used in oral surgery. The systematic presentation of the techniques with detailed demonstrations on acrylic and animal models makes it very easy to understand and practice these techniques, enabling beginners to not only tie single button sutures but also use different suture techniques correctly in their daily work with patients.

I hope both that readers enjoy this book and learn the different suture techniques for use with their patients and that the authors receive positive feedback from their audience.

In long-standing friendship,
Michael Stimmelmayr

Preface

No matter how well a surgical procedure is performed, its outcome is ultimately dependent upon precise wound closure with the correct suturing material and technique. As oral surgical procedures have evolved from macroscopic techniques to microsurgical approaches, suturing techniques, needle sizes, and thread materials have also changed. As a result, selecting the appropriate suture material and method can be confusing for experienced and novice surgeons alike.

This book is a concise resource for understanding the myriad suturing options available to dentists today. The authors have made every effort to include recently developed suturing concepts pertinent to both conventional oral surgery and oral microsurgery. Step-by-step drawings, with accompanying photographs of the techniques performed on an animal model, can be used as easy-to-follow exercises for practice at home. Once the suturing techniques are mastered on a model, they can be readily applied with confidence in a clinical setting.

The final chapter discusses the management of complications encountered during and after surgery. No matter your experience level, you can expect occasional complications, and this section prepares you for those occasions.

Although this book will help prepare you to achieve exceptional surgical outcomes, it is only a guide and a compass. As Sir William Osler once said, "to study medicine without books is to sail an uncharted sea, while to study medicine only from books is not to go to sea at all."

Edward P. Allen

Authors

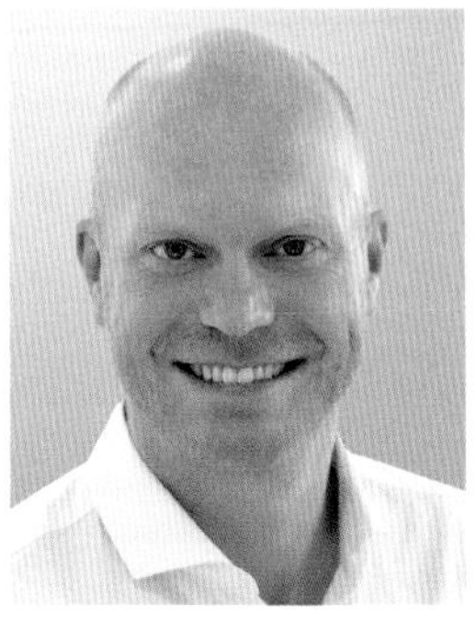

Dr Stephan Beuer, MSc, studied dentistry in Regensburg from 1997 to 2003. After 2 years of preparation in a general dental practice, he completed his specialist training as an oral surgeon in an oral and maxillofacial surgery practice. In 2006 he completed his doctorate under Prof Dr Michael Christgau. Dr Beuer earned his master of science (MSc) degree in orthodontics at the end of 2009. At the beginning of 2010, he opened the Münchnerau practice clinic in Landshut together with Dr Christian A. Kaes. His main areas of treatment are hard and soft tissue augmentation, periodontal surgery, and implantology. He works exclusively as a surgeon. Dr Beuer is also a speaker and author as well as a member of the "New Group" and various other scientific societies.

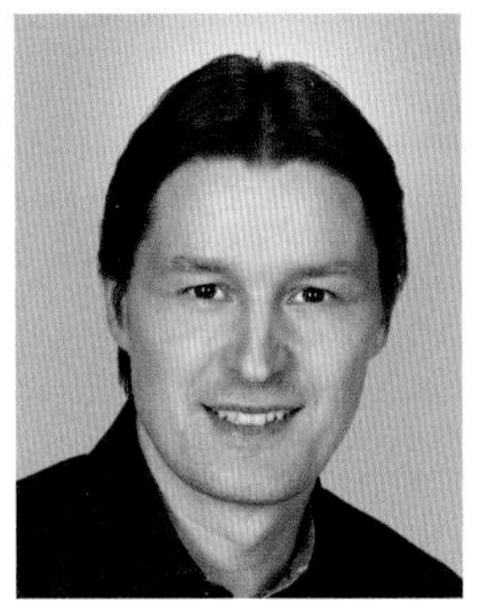

Dr Martin Stangl studied dentistry at the University of Regensburg, Germany, from 2001 to 2007. In 2009, he completed his doctorate under Prof Dr Gottfried Schmalz in dental conservation. Since the beginning of his preparatory period, Dr Stangl has been working with Prof Dr Michael Stimmelmayr in Cham, with whom he founded a joint practice in 2011. In addition to surgical procedures, his main areas of practice are prosthetic and reconstructive dentistry.

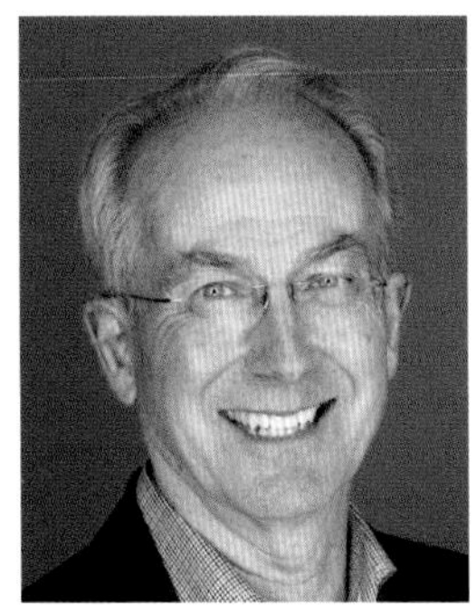

Edward P. Allen, DDS, PhD has served as president of the American Academy of Esthetic Dentistry, the American Academy of Restorative Dentistry, and the American Academy of Periodontology Foundation. He is the recipient of the Master Clinician Award from the American Academy of Periodontology, the President's Award for Excellence in Dental Education from the American Academy of Esthetic Dentistry, and the Saul Schluger Award for Excellence in Diagnosis and Treatment Planning. In 2019, he was honored with the AAP Gold Medal Award, the highest award bestowed by the Academy. Currently, he serves on the editorial boards of the Journal of Esthetic and Restorative Dentistry, the Journal of Periodontology, and the International Journal of Periodontics and Restorative Dentistry. Dr Allen is founder of the Center for Advanced Dental Education in Dallas, an educational facility where he teaches surgical technique courses. He has over 100 publications and has presented numerous lectures and surgical demonstrations worldwide.

Table of Contents

1. Introduction

"I'll be done in a minute. I'll just do a quick sew up!"

Unfortunately, this sentence is heard far too often. Appropriate wound closure complements a surgical procedure as a final step and thus represents a *sine qua non*.

Every complex procedure, especially when it includes augmentation, is followed by a no less complex and time-consuming wound closure; otherwise there is no certainty of a good and predictable result. Sustainability in particular plays a major role. An initial wound closure that loosens due to excessive tension or due to the shape of the graft, resulting in wound dehiscence, is extremely unpleasant for both the patient and the surgeon. It is not uncommon for such a complication to be associated with the loss of the graft and ultimate failure.

Sensitive handling of hard and soft tissue as well as primary and tension-free wound closure are absolutely essential for tissue healing. It is therefore quite clear that the preparation of the flap and the tension-free wound closure need to be given as much time and care as the rest of the procedure. In short, wound closure is the most important part of every surgical procedure!

This book is intended to introduce the reader step by step to high-quality suturing in dental surgery. Particular emphasis is placed on teaching the basic suturing techniques. For more specialized suturing techniques, the reader is referred to the appropriate periodontal surgery books. This book is intended to serve the practitioner as an uncomplicated handbook that can be consulted at any time.

The individual chapters are structured in such a way that first an informational box provides indications and other basic information for a particular suture. Subsequently, the suture techniques are illustrated on acrylic and animal (pig ear) models.

2. Suture Instruments

2.1 Needle

Each suture material must be paired with a suitable needle. There is a wide range of needles to choose from in the field of dental surgery. Today's manufacturers ensure that needles meet the requirements in terms of sharpness, good piercing ability, elasticity, and bending strength, as well as sterility.

When selecting needles, some parameters have to be considered. Let us first look at the basic structure of a needle (Fig 1). Of clinical importance are, above all, the shape of the bend, the needle tip, the needle eye, and the needle code.

2.1.1 Bend

The bend is given as a fraction of a full circle. In dental surgery, 3/8- and 1/2-circle needles with an arc length between 9 and 18 mm are most often used (Fig 2). Straight needle shapes are only used extremely rarely and are suitable for interdental sutures, for example.

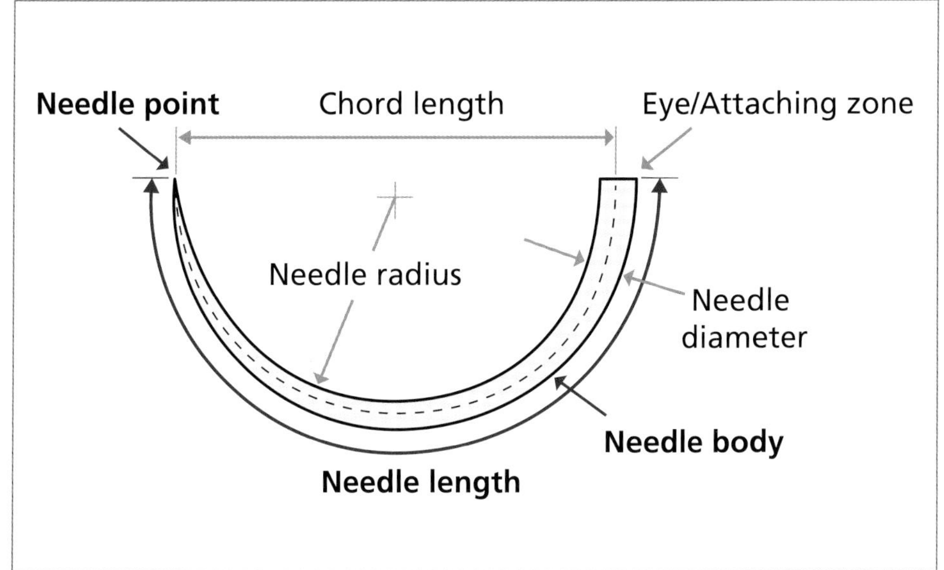

1 Needle structure.

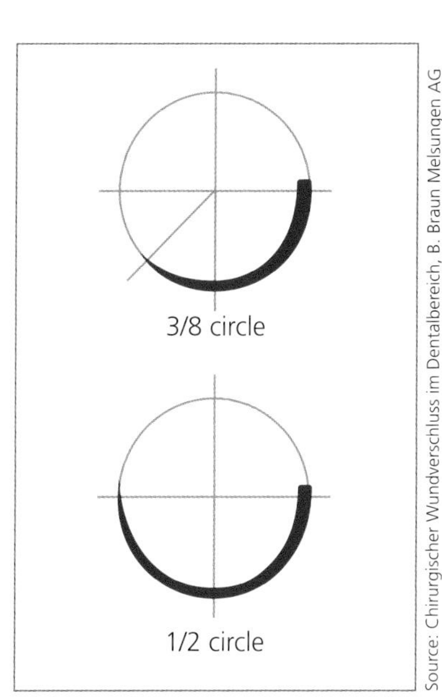

2 The most popular needle shapes in oral surgery are 3/8- and 1/2-circle.

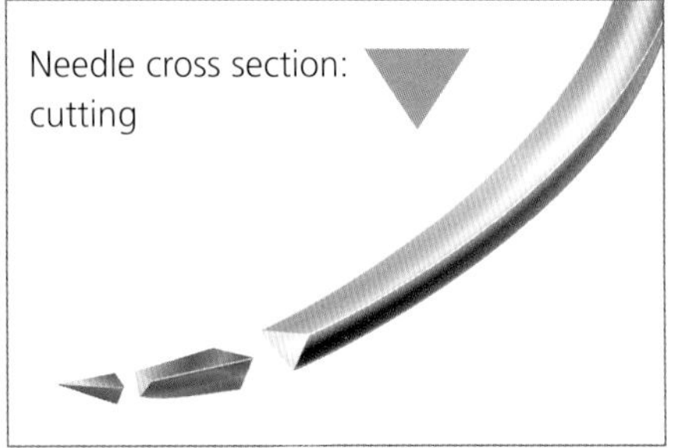

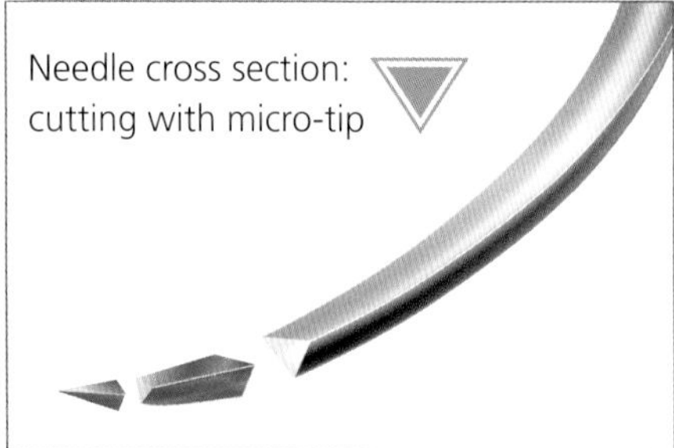

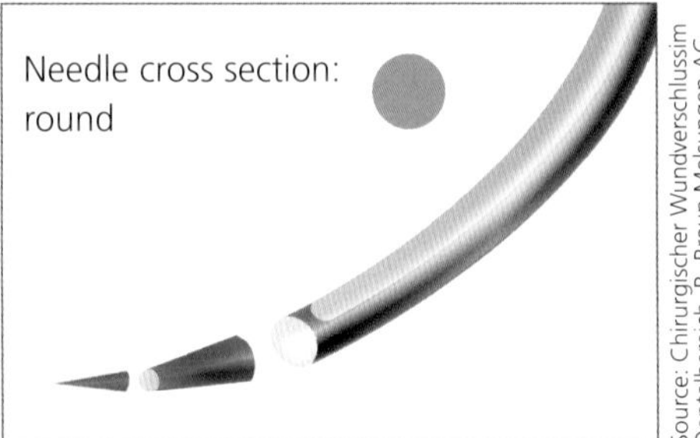

Source: Chirurgischer Wundverschlussim Dentalbereich, B. Braun Melsungen AG

3 **The triangular, externally cutting needle body is indicated for suturing tough tissue. The three cutting edges extend the entire length of the needle and allow optimal piercing ability with a reliable, cosmetic result.**

4 **The cutting micro-tip of this slim precision needle is hand sharpened and allows very good tissue penetration, very fine sutures in attached tissue, and very good cosmetic results with minimal trauma.**

5 **The round body of the needle tapers to a fine, sharp needle point. Round-bodied needles only pierce the tissue, they do not cut. Therefore, they are well suited for sutures in soft tissue.**

2.1.2 Needle tip

The needle tip extends from the sharpened end to the point at which the needle reaches its full cross section. We distinguish:

- The triangular cutting needle (Fig 3)
- The micro-tip cutting needle (Fig 4)
- The round needle (Fig 5)

Note that although there are various other needle shapes and tips, they do not play a prominent role in dental surgery.

The choice of needle should be based on the indication because the piercing behavior is very different in connective tissue than in keratinized gingiva.

2.1.3 Eye/Attaching zone (connection between needle and thread)

The type of connection between the needle and thread is important. In this context, the terms *traumatic* and *atraumatic* are often used.

In traumatic suturing, the needle and thread consist of two parts connected by the eye of the needle. The eye of the needle can be either closed (as with sewing needles) or open to allow the thread to be hooked in. A crucial problem is the incongruent size relationship between the needle and thread, which causes trauma when penetrating the tissue (hence the term *traumatic*). In addition, bacteria can be carried deep into the niches between the needle and thread. This can impair wound healing. Fortunately, traumatic suture materials are hardly ever used anymore.

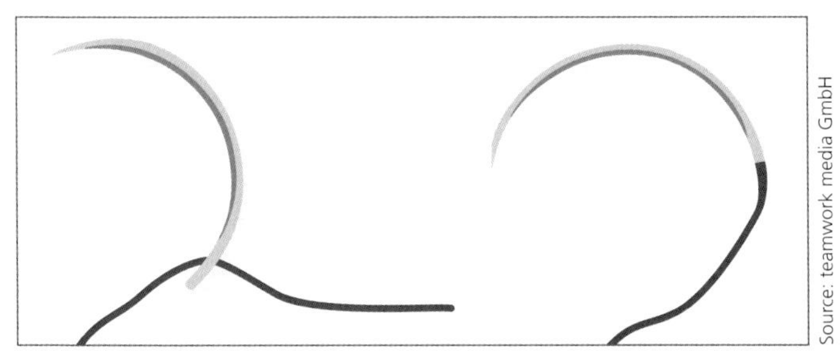

Source: teamwork media GmbH

6 **Difference between traumatic (left) and atraumatic (right) needles.**

Today, the atraumatic suture is the method of choice and has largely replaced the traumatic suture in oral surgery. A swaged needle has no eye, but rather the thread is attached to a hollow end. The connection between the needle and the thread appears to be seamless because one end of the thread is attached to the distal end of the needle by a cylindrical part (hollow-cylinder system) or a throat (flange system). Unfortunately, it is still very difficult to achieve the ideal 1:1 ratio between the needle and thread all the time.

2.1.4 Needle code

The needle code provides information on the size and condition of the needle and consists of a letter-number combination (Fig 7). The first letter indicates the needle anatomy; the second letter marks the shape of the needle body. If a third or fourth letter follows, they refer to special features of the needle. The number after the letters indicates the needle length in stretched form (arc length) in millimeters (mm). Figure 8 shows a package with the needle code DS12.

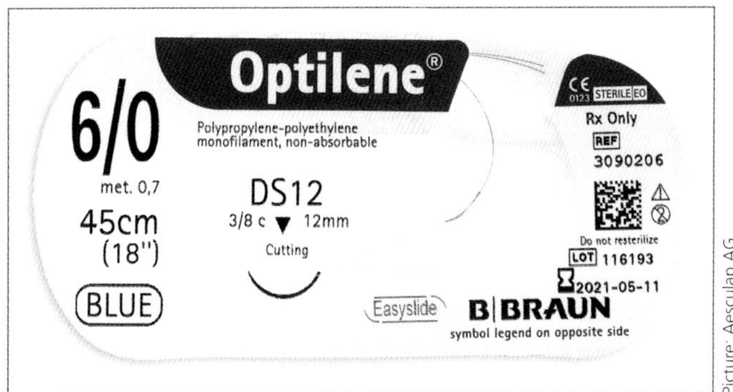

Picture: Aesculap AG

8 Example of a monofilament, nonabsorbable thread of strength 6/0 (D = 3/8-circle, S = cutting needle, 12 = arc length in mm). For some suture suppliers, the needle designations do not allow direct reference to the needle.

Important

- In dental surgery, mainly 3/8- and 1/2-circle needle shapes are used.
- Only atraumatic needles should be used.
- The needle code includes needle curvature, body, tip, and length.

Needle curvature	Needle body	Needle tip	Needle length	Additional information
S 1/8-circle	**R round body**	**T trocar tip**	**The numbers indicate the distance from needle tip to end in mm, measured at the outer curvature of the needle.**	
V 1/4-circle	**S cutting**	N blunt tip		
D 3/8-circle	L lancet	S cutting tip/inside		s strong needle body ss very strong needle body
H 1/2-circle	SP spatula	C short cutting tip		
F 5/8-circle		**MP micro-tip/precision**		
G straight		m micro-needle		
P progressive				

Source: Chirurgischer Wundverschluss im Dentalbereich, B. Braun Melsungen AG

7 The needle code: The areas marked in dark gray reflect the dental priorities. An example of this can be seen in Figure 8 (DS12).

2.2 Thread

In addition to the needle, the thread is an essential component of the suture material. Surgical suture material can be classified according to the criteria of absorbability, thread structure, and thread strength.

2.2.1 Absorbability

The most important distinction is between absorbable and nonabsorbable sutures (Fig 9). Absorbability is the calculated and intended dissolvability of a suture in living human or animal tissue.

In the case of absorbable filaments, polymers of glycolic or lactic acid and polydioxanones are mainly used today. Their degradation takes place via hydrolysis, with the end products being CO_2 and H_2O. This avoids the occurrence of superfluous inflammatory reactions. The data on the absorption time should be regarded as approximate because many factors (eg, mechanical forces, thread strength, tissue type, local infections, general condition of the patient) cannot be specified exactly and may vary considerably.

Indications for absorbable sutures range from suturing with multilayer techniques to use in very young, apprehensive patients and/or patients with infectious disease or multiple morbidities.

Nonabsorbable suture material is used for all other indications. The tension resistance should be maintained for at least 60 days. Synthetic materials such as polyamide polymers (nylon), polyester fibers made of polyethylene terephthalate, and propylene polymers and polyvinyl polymers are mainly used. These are synthetic polymers whose quality can be kept consistent.

Silk is another nonabsorbable natural multifilament suture material but should no longer be used in dental surgery due to its capillarity and the associated bacterial load on the tissue. In the case of monofilament sutures, the inner space is completely closed, and thus any form of capillarity is excluded. This property allows the threads to be left in place for a longer period of time.

As a general rule, it is better to err toward leaving sutures in place for too long rather than not long enough in the case of complex surgical procedures. Because these materials do not react with the environment, they can be removed without complications even after being in place for weeks.

Catgut—a natural suture material made from the intestinal tissue of sheep or cattle—is no longer used because of the risk of prion transmission, among other reasons. Only synthetically produced materials are used today. Synthetic suture materials

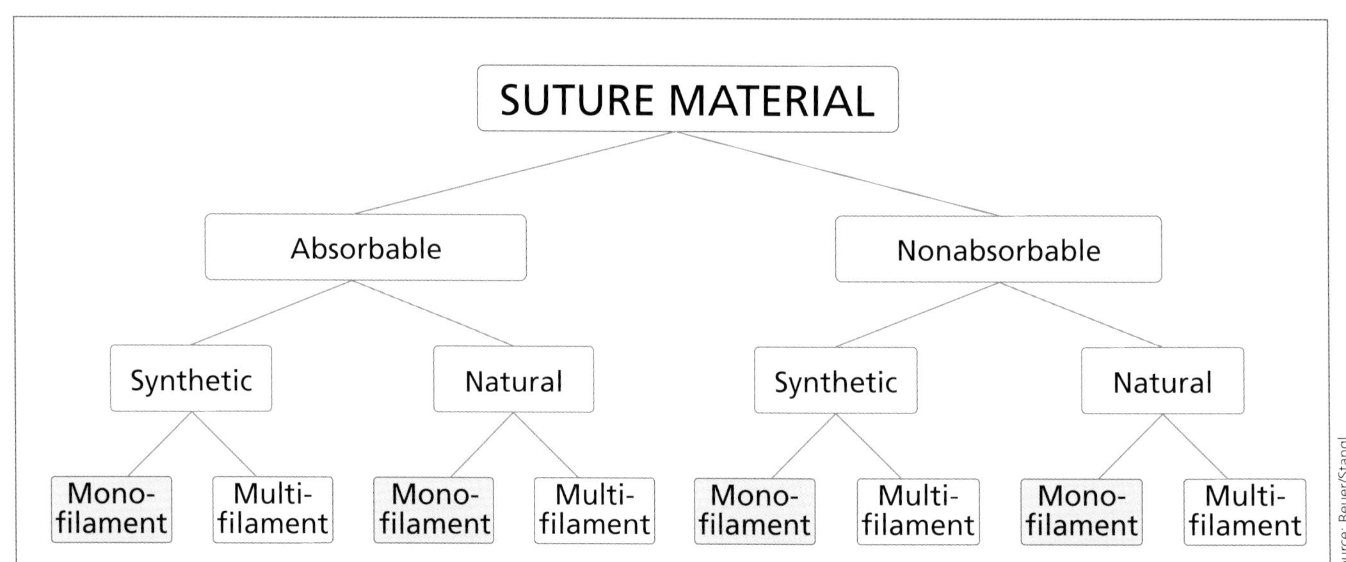

9 **Breakdown of suture materials according to absorbability, origin, and thread structure.**

offer consistent quality, whereas natural suture materials exhibit variation in their physical properties.

In principle, it is important to remove nonabsorbable suture material; otherwise, a foreign body reaction with connective tissue entrapment of the suture can occur. In the context of wound healing, this can have a detrimental effect after removal of the suture.

2.2.2 Thread structure

Another important feature of suture materials is the structure of the filaments. Monofilament materials can be differentiated from pseudomonofilament and multifilament materials (Fig 10).

Monofilament sutures consist of one piece and are the most popular suture material in dental surgery. They have the best properties for gliding through the tissue, and the smooth, closed surface prevents any capillarity, which means they cannot absorb and pass on water in the filaments. On the negative side, monofilament filaments have a high elastic memory. That is, the force restoring it to its original position is high, and the knot can open more easily. This elastic memory is the highest in nylon. In addition, monofilament threads are sensitive to external damage, for example, when gripping the thread with instruments. Nonabsorbable expanded polytetrafluoroethylene (ePTFE) monofilament sutures have the best lubricity.

Multifilament suture material consists of a large number of individual threads or filaments of identical thickness that can be braided or twisted. This increases physical properties such as strength, elasticity, and flexibility and thus significantly improves the knot strength.

On the other hand, multifilament threads have a rough surface, making it more difficult for them to pass through the tissue, which has a negative effect on the friction behavior. Likewise, multifilament sutures have greater capillarity, which favors the adhesion of bacteria. A classic example of a natural multifilament suture is silk, which should no longer be used in oral surgery. The lubricity of silk is significantly worse compared to monofilament suture materials.

Pseudomonofilament suture materials are coated or sheathed multifilament materials. The coating smooths the rough surface, facilitating passage through tissue and reducing capillarity. Thanks to this measure, the advantages of monofilament suture materials are obtained while the disadvantages are reduced, ie, the knot fit is tighter, and the threads are less wiry and stiff. Dyeing the suture material allows easier identification of the suture in the wound area.

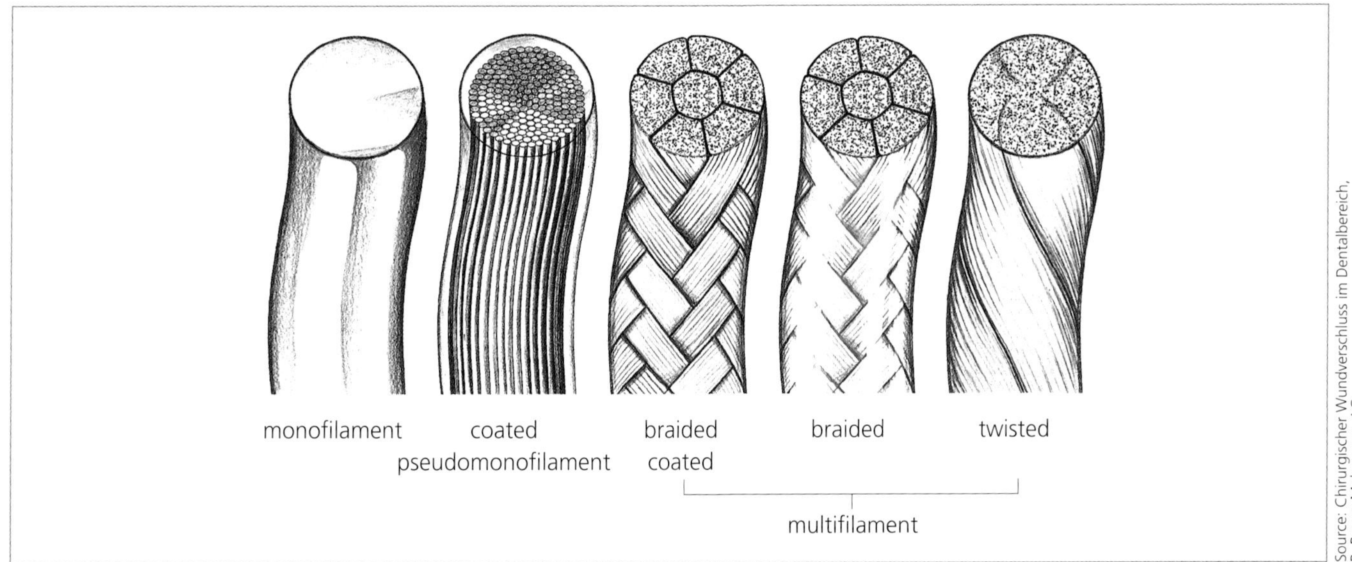

10 Thread structure as a classification criterion: monofilament versus multifilament.

2.2.3 Thread strength

The specific properties of the thread are determined not only by the material and the thread structure but also by its strength and cross section (Fig 11). The strength classification is regulated, and there are basically two different systems for designating strength.

The first is the metric strength designation of the European Pharmacopoeia (EP). The diameter designation is metric, and the filament diameter is given in increments of 0.1 mm. On the other hand, there is the classification according to the United States Pharmacopoeia (USP). In this classification, the thread strength designation is arbitrary and not directly related to the thread diameter.

Although classification according to EP would be more rational, the USP classification is predominantly used today. In dental surgery, suture material of strength 4/0 to 7/0 is recommended for surgical procedures.

The rule is: As thin as necessary and as thick as possible. As thin as necessary means that the tissue must not be traumatized or the blood supply cut off. As thick as possible means that thicker thread makes it easier for the practitioner to place and remove the sutures.

Important

- Suture materials are classified into absorbable versus non-absorbable and natural versus synthetic materials.
- The thread structure, the thread thickness, and the material determine the tensile strength and knotting properties.
- The smaller the thread diameter, the lower the tissue damage but also the lower the tensile strength.
- It is better to leave the suture material in situ for too long rather than not long enough.

Thread Strength		
Metric	USP	Diameter (in mm)
0.01	12/0	0.001–0.009
0.1	11/0	0.010–0.019
0.2	10/0	0.020–0.029
0.3	9/0	0.030–0.039
0. 4	8/0	0.040–0.049
0.5	7/0	0.050–0.069
0.7	6/0	0.070–0.099
1	5/0	0.100–0.149
1.5	4/0	0.150–0.199
2	3/0	0.200–0.249
2.5–3	2/0	0.250–0.349
3.5	0	0.350–0,399
4	1	0.400–0.499
5	2	0.500–0.599
6	3	0.600–0.699
7	5	0.700–0.799

Source: Chirurgischer Wundverschluss im Dentalbereich, B. Braun Melsungen AG

11 Conversion chart for thread strength classification.

2.3 Needle holder

The task of the needle holder is to fix the needle and thread and guide them safely through the tissue during suturing. A distinction is made between two different types of needle holders:

- Needle holder with a lock (eg, Matthieu, Mayo-Hegar)
- Needle holder without a lock (eg, Axhausen, Toennis)—extremely rarely used

Needle holders with a ratchet locking system securely fix the needle between the jaw surfaces. This allows easy guidance of the needle through the tissue, especially in surgical areas that are difficult to access. In contrast, there are needle holders without a ratchet locking mechanism, which require the surgeon to apply pressure to fix the needle.

Both types of needle holders are available in various lengths, widths, and branch sizes. Each operator must choose from the variety of needle holders available according to his or her preferences.

Needle holders are highly specific, just like needle and thread. Needles with a diameter of 3/0, 4/0, or 5/0 require large, robust jaw surfaces. For microsurgical or periodontal surgical procedures with a suture thickness of 6/0 or 7/0 or more, a microsurgical needle holder with delicate and fine jaw surfaces (Castroviejo needle holder) is required. Microsurgical needle holders should be held in the hand like a pen. The rest of the needle holder also has specific modifications to allow very thin needles and sutures to be easily guided through the tissue.

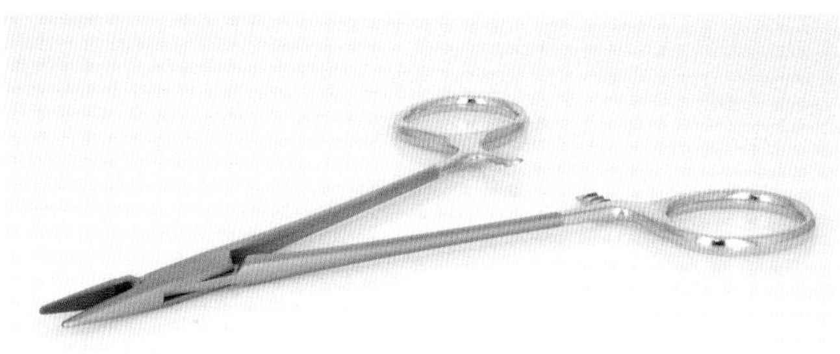

12 **Baby-Crile-Wood needle holder (BM013R from Aesculap Dental).**

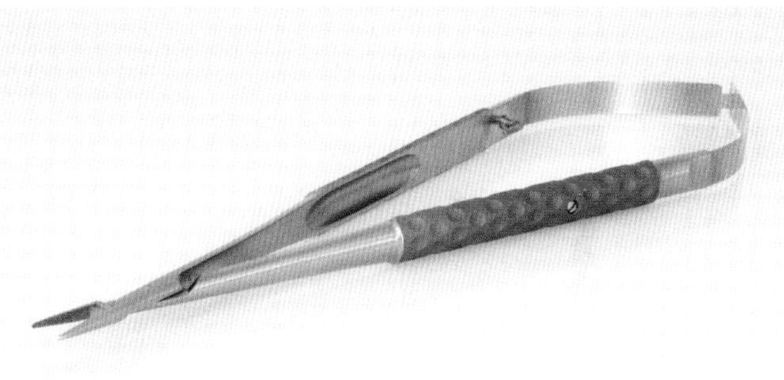

13 **Castroviejo microsurgical needle holder (FD258R, Diadust from Aesculap Dental, with diamond powder–coated working ends for suture material of thickness 6/0 to 9/0).**

2 Pictures: teamwork media GmbH

2.4 Tweezers

Tweezers (or forceps) are a type of grasping instrument and are divided into dental, surgical (Fig 14), and anatomical depending on their function. The functions of these instruments are the insertion and removal of materials into the surgical area and the fixation of the tissue during suturing. While dental tweezers have a curved working end, anatomical and surgical tweezers have a straight working end. For a secure hold and for moving tissue, surgical tweezers have two teeth at the working end, which interlock perfectly when closed. In contrast, dental and anatomical tweezers have a transversely serrated working end without teeth. It should be noted that the teeth on surgical tweezers can traumatize the tissue during fixation.

In the case of microsurgical and periodontal plastic surgical procedures where 6/0 and smaller needles are used, the microsurgical tweezers (or forceps) have delicate working ends with diamond powder coating rather than serrated surfaces to minimize damage to delicate tissues. An additional use of microsurgical forceps is in the capturing of the smaller needles in microsurgical procedures. For this purpose, the jaws may be lightly roughened, or diamond dusted rather than transversely serrated to improve grip on the suture (Fig 15). Serrated jaws are too coarse for microsurgery and are more likely to injure the suture and bur the needle leading to trauma to the delicate tissues.

2.5 Scissors

Scissors are used in oral surgery for cutting suture material and suture removal and also for cutting tissue. Straight or slightly curved scissors with a pointed working end are used for cutting suture material and preparing tissue.

Absorbable sutures should be shortened as much as possible to avoid unnecessary absorption of suture material. In contrast, nonabsorbable sutures should be shortened to a length of 4 to 6 mm. This avoids unpleasant poking of the suture ends and facilitates suture removal.

Microsurgical scissors are commonly used for microsurgical and periodontal surgical procedures in the same way as microsurgical needle holders and forceps (Fig 16).

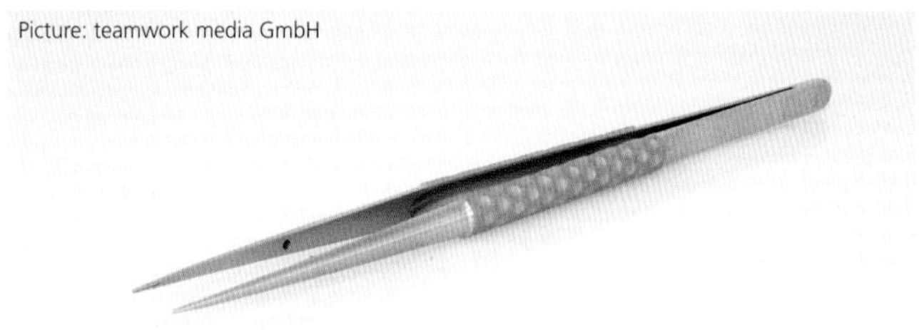

14 **Cooley atraumatic micro forceps (DX303R from Aesculap Dental).**

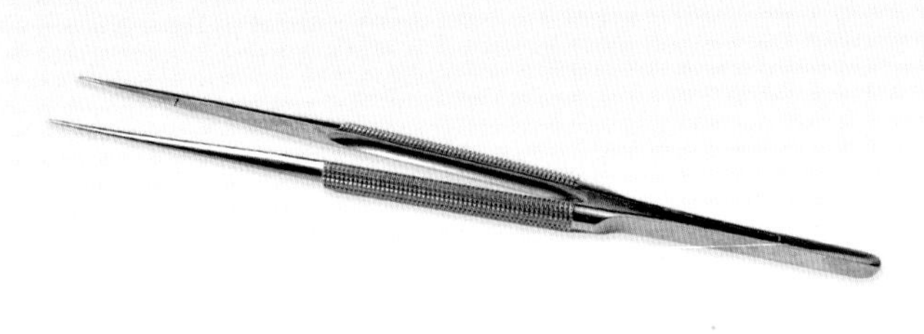

15 **Microsurgical forceps (Micro Dressing Forcep 8-905DD from Hu-Friedy).**

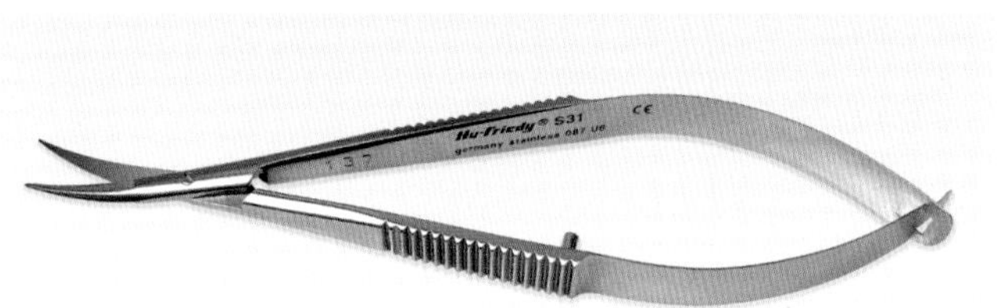

16 **Micro Castroviejo scissors (S31 from Hu-Friedy).**

3. General Rules of Suturing in Dental Surgery

Suturing is the most important step of any surgical intervention in the oral cavity because it determines predictable success or failure in almost all cases. The purpose of suturing is the appropriate adaptation of the wound edges during the healing phase.

It is important to use the correct instruments. The use of the appropriate needle holder, tweezers, and scissors is crucial when suturing (see chapter 2).

When starting each suture after the needle has been picked up, the soft tissue of the movable flap is first pierced with the needle and then joined to the fixed soft tissue. Opinions regarding the ideal holding position of the needle holder vary slightly. The grip of the needle for 6/0 and 7/0 suture material should be at the midpoint of the needle to avoid bending of the needle that occurs when the needle is gripped near the jaw of the needleholder. The needle should penetrate perpendicular to the tissue. Alternatively, the needle holder may hold the needle at a ratio of 2/3 (distance from the needle tip to the jaw of the needle holder) to 1/3 (distance between the jaws of the needle holder to the needle-thread transition). This is to prevent the needle tip from being bent or otherwise damaged due to lack of control (which occurs when the needle is picked up too far from the tip) and also to prevent the action radius from being too restricted (which occurs when the needle is picked up too close to the needle tip). In principle, the needle insertions should be done in the attached gingiva to prevent scarring. To prevent tearing of the tissue, grasping at least 3 to 5 mm from the tissue margins is essential. For oral surgery, the authors recommend the use of monofilament suture materials, which should have a USP strength of 4/0 to 7/0, depending on the area of application. In soft tissue surgery, especially in periodontal plastic surgery, the use of 6/0 and 7/0 sutures is recommended. With thinner sutures, the added benefits fail to compensate for the extra effort required. For the classic surgical knot, a 2-1-1* knot is sufficient for sutures thicker than 6/0. For sutures size 6/0 and thinner, the authors recommend tying a 3-2-1, 3-1-2, or 3-1-1 knot, as this largely prevents the knot from coming loose, especially after the first fixation. The knot should therefore be secured with a series of clockwise and counterclockwise knots.

Tip: Absorbable sutures are advisable for subcutaneous and multilayer sutures, as well as for patients with mental and physical disabilities. Except for these special indications, the monofilament, nonabsorbable suture is the material of choice because of the low tissue reaction.

* The numbers indicate the number of times each knot is thrown over, with the first and third knots tied in the same direction and the second knot tied in the opposite direction.

4. The Surgical Knot: Suture Techniques

Suture Techniques and Their Indications at a Glance

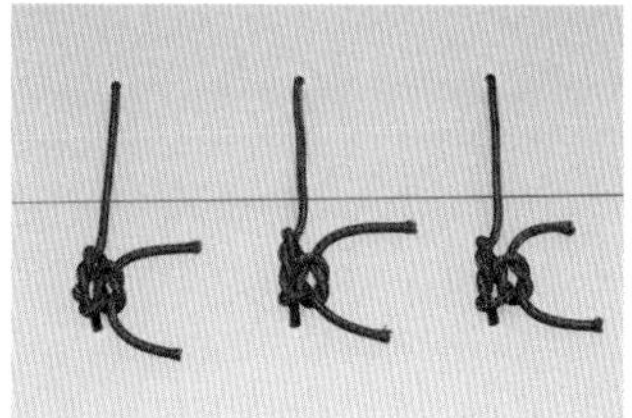

4.1 Single button suture (see p 14)

- Most commonly used suture
- Adaptation of wound edges
- Initial suture for stabilization of complex flaps
- Blood vessel ligation
- Not suitable for relieving tension in flaps

4.2 Mattress suture

- Suitable for relieving tension in flaps
- Active positioning of the flap and wound edges
- Used in extractions and periodontal and implant surgery
- Important for coverage after augmentation
- Important for primary wound closure following, among other things, augmentation procedures

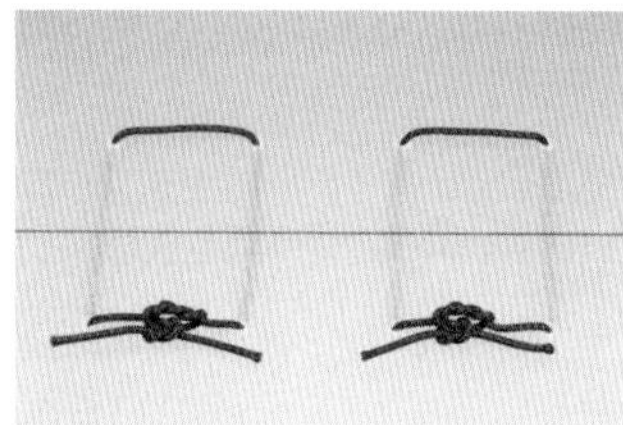

4.2.1 Horizontal mattress suture (see p 22)

- Most important suture for covering defects and after augmentation procedures
- Enables two-dimensional adaptation of the wound edges and stabilization of the flap

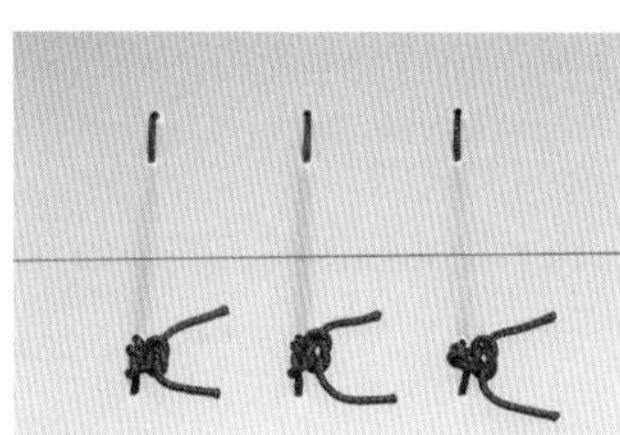

4.2.2 Vertical mattress suture (see p 30)

- Indicated for limited horizontal space conditions (eg, between teeth)

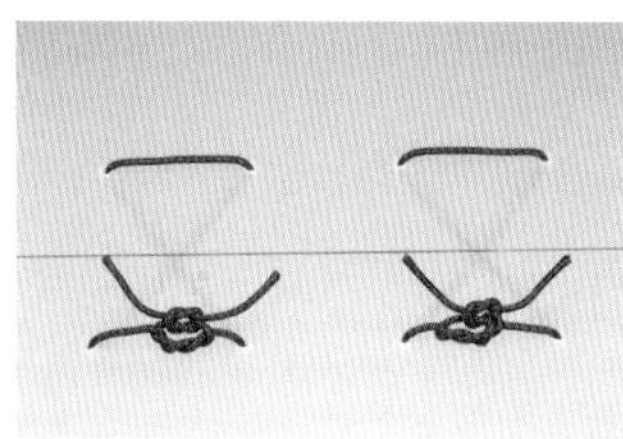

4.2.3 Cross mattress suture (see p 38)

- Used in extractions to stabilize the blood clot and wound edges
- In the case of inhomogeneous alveolar ridge anatomy, used to achieve stable adaptation of the wound margins

4.3 Laurell suture

- Suitable for relieving tension in flaps
- Active positioning of the flap and wound edges
- Used in extractions and periodontal and implant surgery
- Helps with coverage after augmentation procedures
- Helps in the creation of primary wound closure

Note: Also referred to as Laurell-Gottlow suture; combination of mattress and single button sutures.

- Advantage: Saves time compared to the combination of mattress and single button sutures.
- Disadvantages: If part of the thread comes loose, the entire suture comes undone; the position of the single button suture depends on the position of the mattress suture.

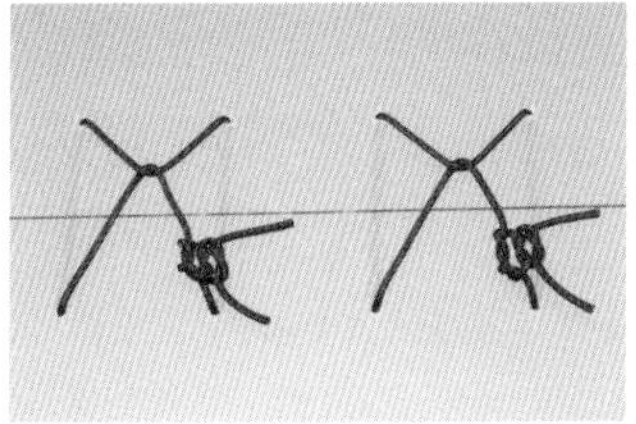

4.3.1 Horizontal Laurell suture (see p 42)

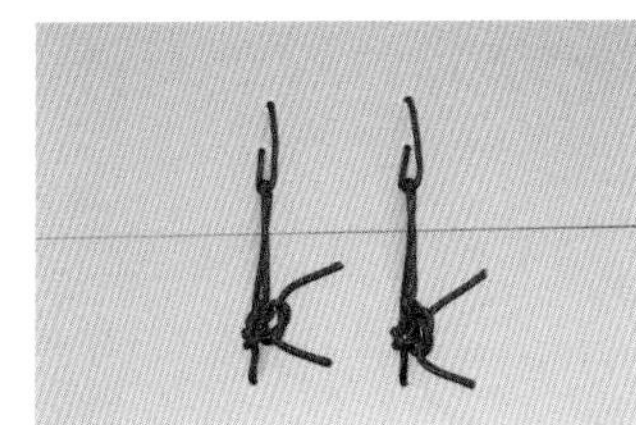

4.3.2 Vertical Laurell suture (see p 50)

4.4 Continuous suture (see p 58)

4.4.1 Simple continuous suture

4.4.2 Continuous interlocking suture

- Closure of long incisions that do not have great esthetic relevance
- For gaping wounds after serial extractions
- In the edentulous ridge
- For repositioning osteotomies in the maxilla

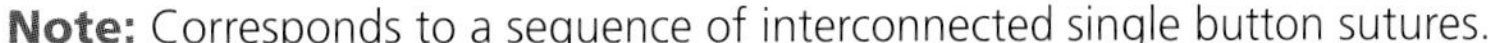

Note: Corresponds to a sequence of interconnected single button sutures.

- Advantage: Saves time compared to single button sutures.
- Disadvantage: If a part of the thread comes loose, the tension of the thread is released in the entire surrounding tissue.

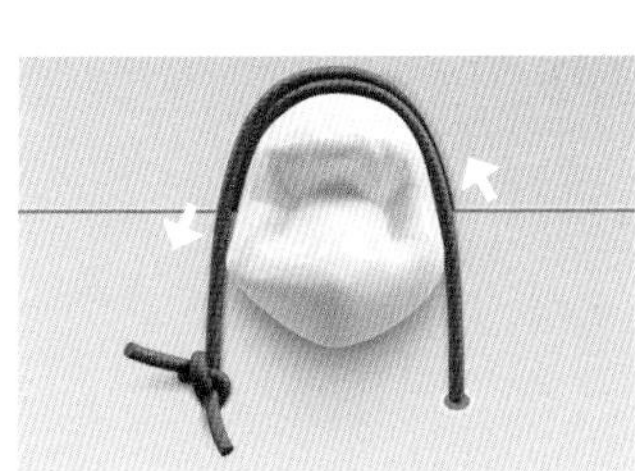

4.5 Simple sling suture (see p 66)

- Suitable for securing a coronally advanced flap
- Tunneling procedures
- Used in root coverage procedures
- Important for adapting the tissue margin at the CEJ
- Can be used for a single tooth or multiple teeth

4.1 Single button suture

Indications:

- Most commonly used suture
- Adaptation of wound edges
- Initial suture for stabilization of complex flaps
- Blood vessel ligation
- Not suitable for relieving tension in flaps

White arrow: Beginning of thread
Gray arrow: End of thread

3–5 mm
3–5 mm
Short thread end (about 15–20 mm)

1 The first step is to pierce the mobilized flap from the outside. **2** The thread penetrates the second flap from the inside. **3** Ensure sufficient distance to the wound edges (approximately 3 to 5 mm). **4** Now the knot is formed. The long end is looped twice around the needle holder.

Schematic representation

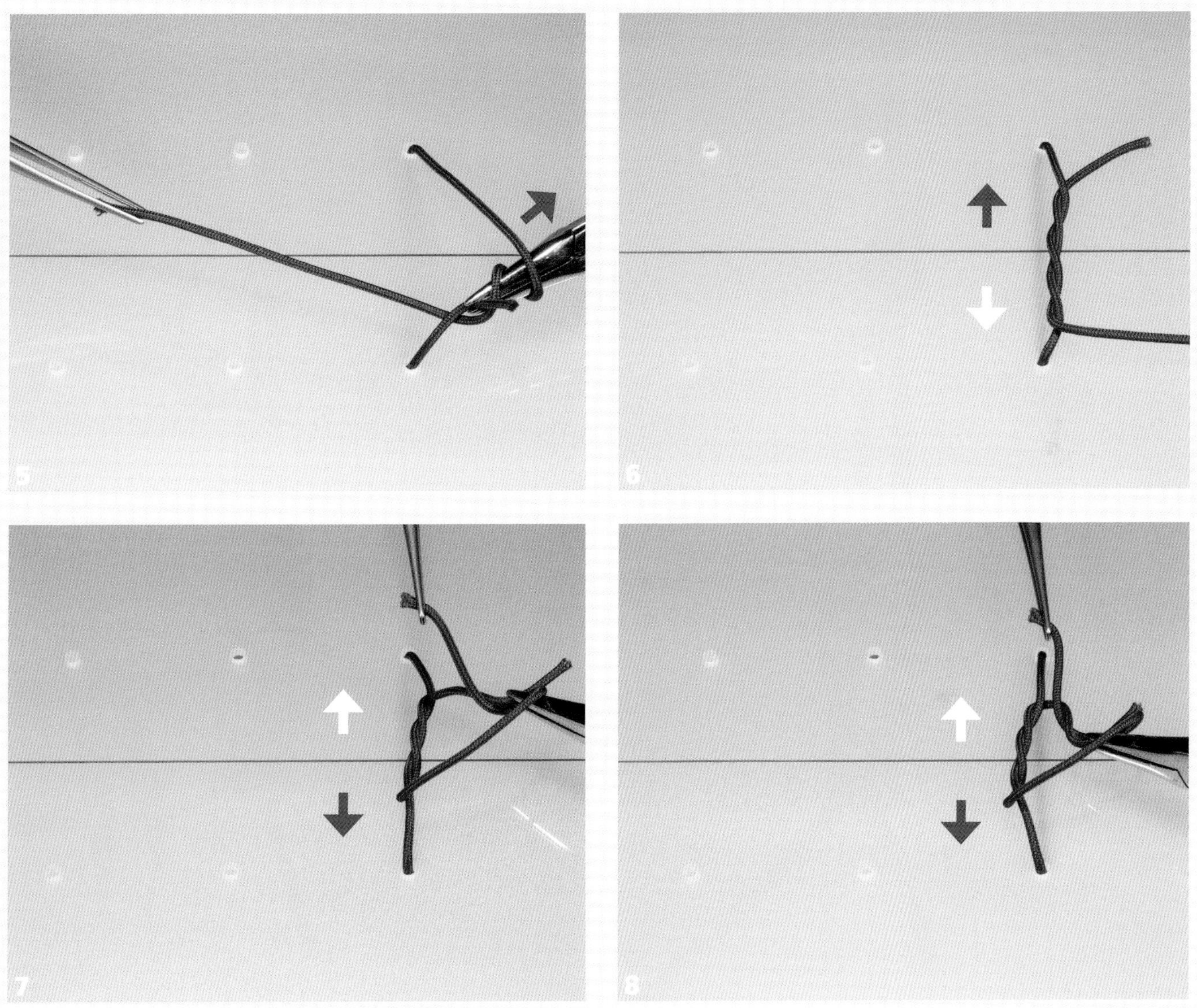

5 The short end is grasped with the needle holder and pulled through. **6** The knot is tightened and should take a stable position. It lies straight and shows a spiral pattern. **7** Another knot is made in the opposite direction with a throw. **8** The knot is tightened again.

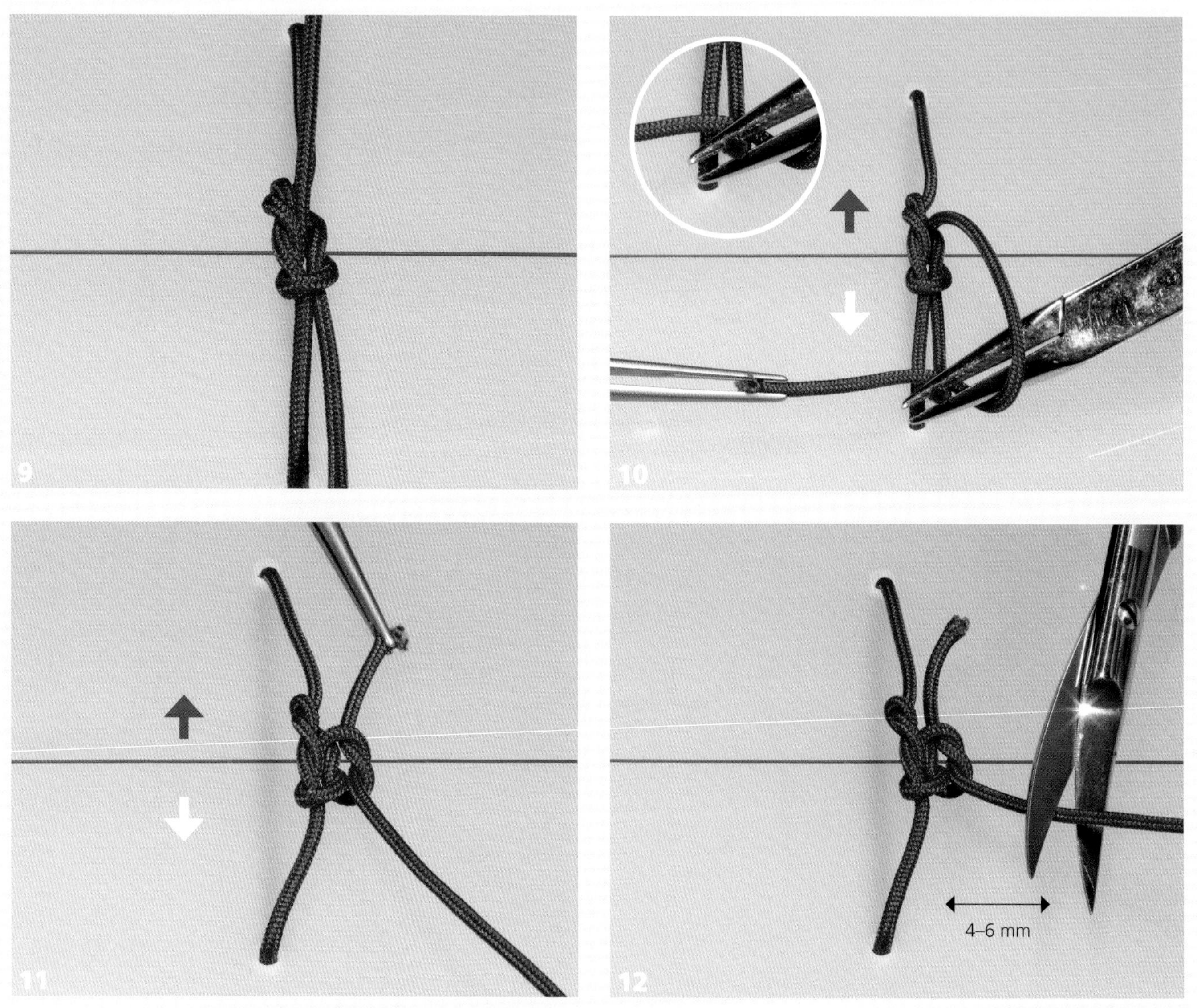

9 It is ensured that the knot can no longer open. **10** Another safety knot in the same direction as the first knot finalizes the surgical knot. **11** The third knot is fixed, changing the forceps from the long to the short end. **12** The knot is cut with the scissors to a thread length of 4 to 6 mm.

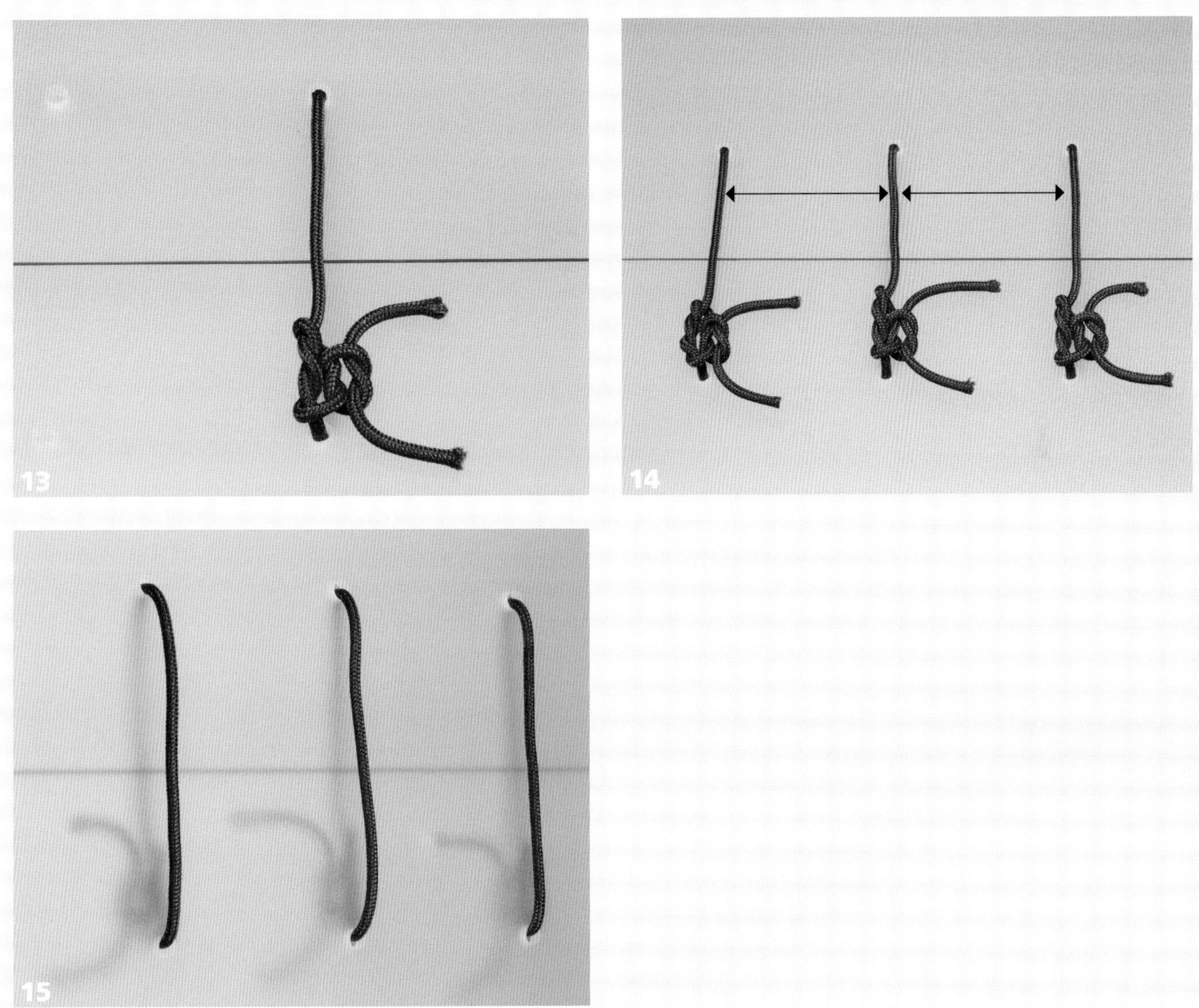

13 The knot should be located to the side of the wound gap, preferably in the area of the keratinized gingiva. **14** Overview of three adjacent single button sutures, which ideally have an equal distance between them. **15** Overview of the single button sutures "from below" (tissue side).

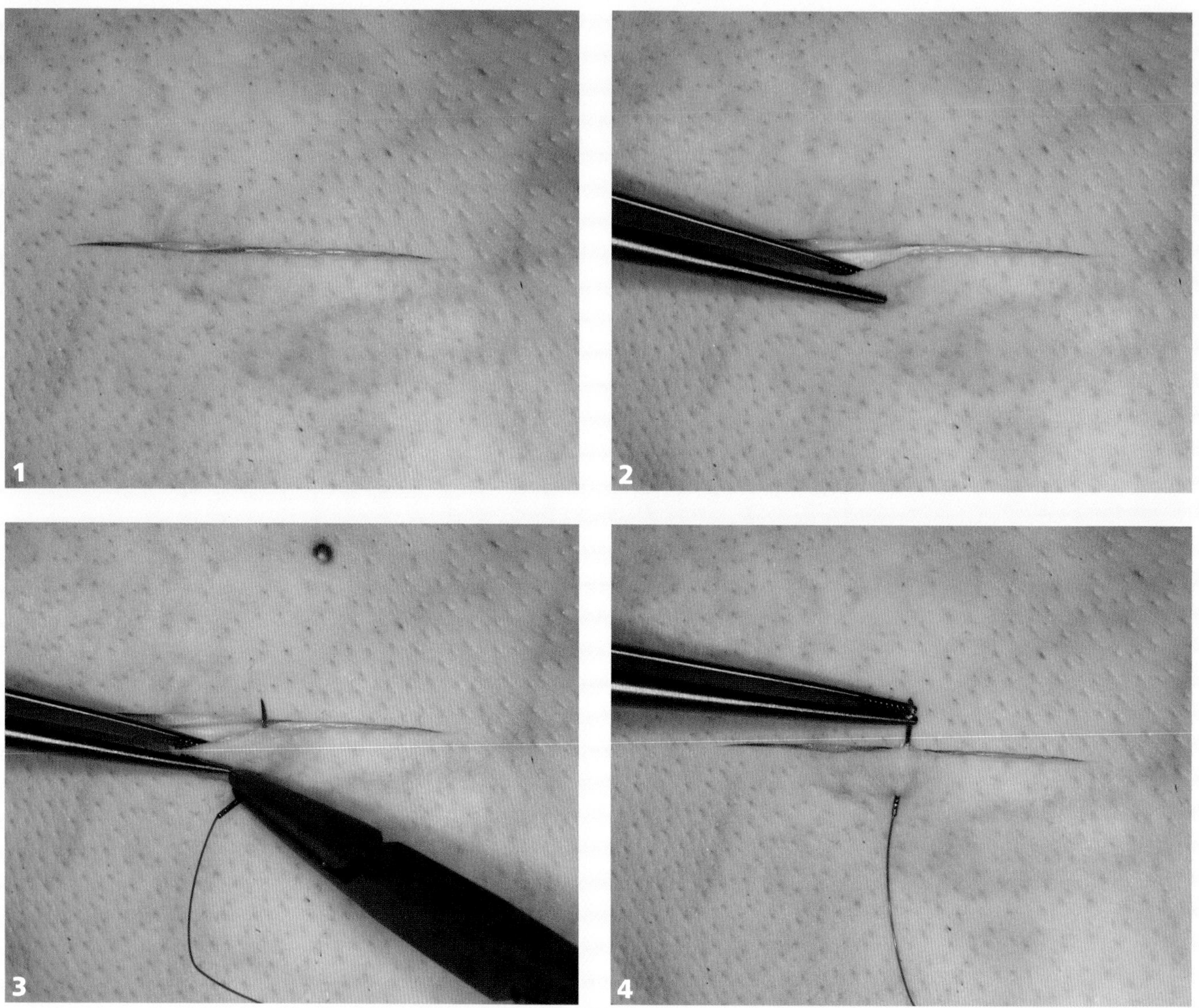

1 Incision on the pig's ear. **2** The flap is grasped with the forceps, thus forming a deliberate abutment to the pressure of the needle. **3** The flap is penetrated from the outside to the inside with sufficient distance to the wound margin. The needle is guided through the tissue. It is picked up at a ratio of 2/3 to 1/3. **4** The needle tip is picked up again after penetration of the tissue has been completed.

Representation on the animal model

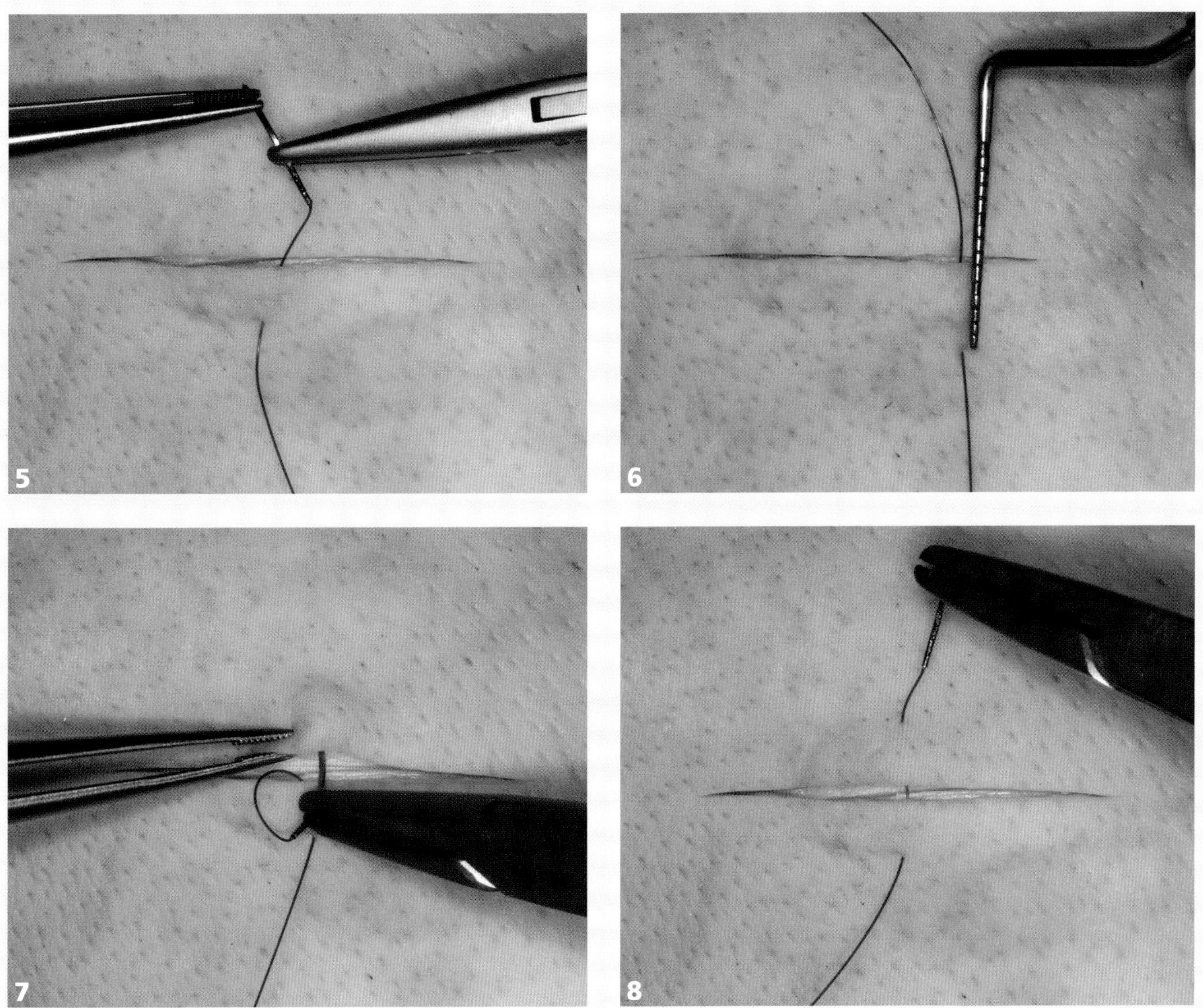

5 The needle is fixed in the ideal position again with the needle holder. **6** The distance of the puncture site from the wound edge should be at least 3 mm. **Caution:** If the tissue is damaged or the distance from the wound edge is too small, the sutures may tear out. **7** The needle penetrates the second flap from the inside to the outside. **8** The needle tip is picked up again with the needle holder. The distance to the wound edge should be the same on both sides of the flap.

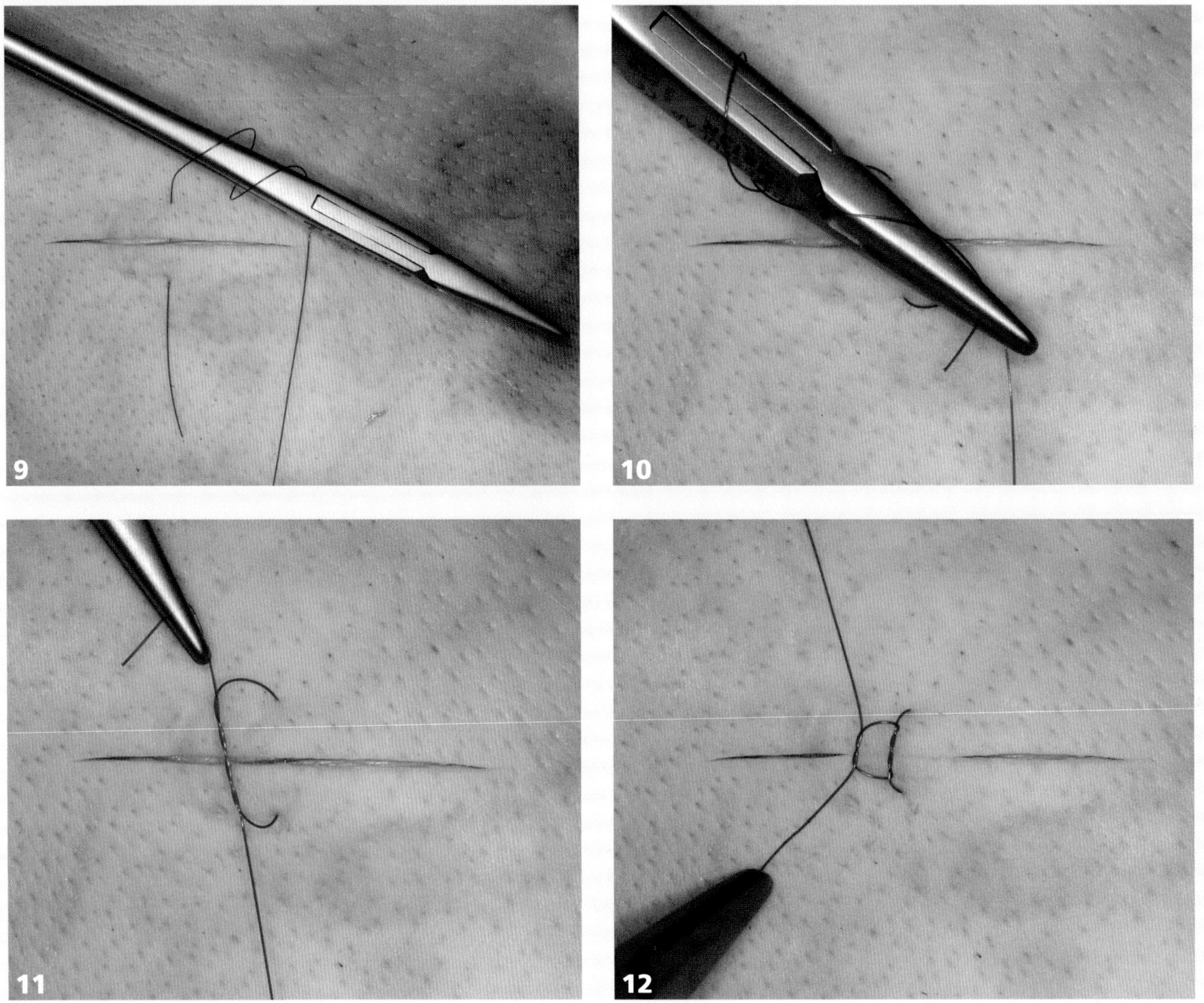

9 Now the knot is formed. The long end is looped twice around the needle holder ... **10** ... and the short end of the thread is picked up with the tip and pulled through. **11** Now the first knot is fixed. The thread should come to lie smooth and in a spiral pattern. **12** Then the second knot is fixed in the opposite direction to the first with a throw (see schematic diagram).

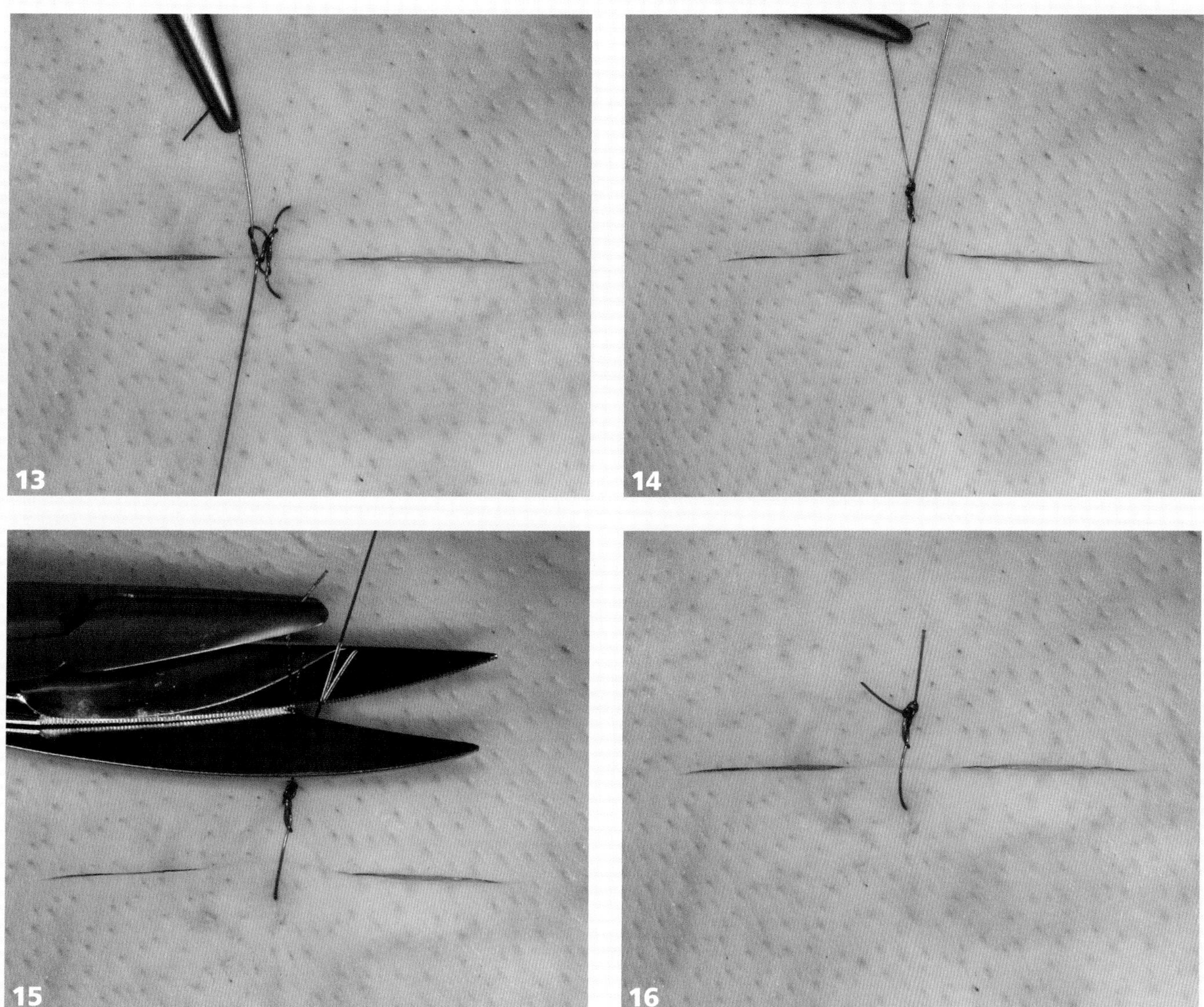

13 Fixing the third knot in the opposite direction to the second knot, also with a throw, finalizes the knot. **14** The knot should be located away from the wound gap (not on the wound gap), preferably in the area of the keratinized gingiva, if present. **15** The ends of the sutures are cut to a length of approximately 4 to 6 mm using scissors. **16** Finished single button suture in place.

4.2 Mattress suture

4.2.1 Horizontal mattress suture

Indications for mattress sutures:

- Suitable for relieving tension in flaps
- Active positioning of the flap and wound edges
- Used in extractions and periodontal and implant surgery
- Important for coverage after augmentation
- Important for the creation of primary wound closure following, among other things, augmentation procedures

Indications for horizontal mattress sutures:

- Most important suture for covering defects and after augmentative procedures
- Enables two-dimensional adaptation of the wound edges and stabilization of the flap

White arrow: Beginning of thread
Gray arrow: End of thread

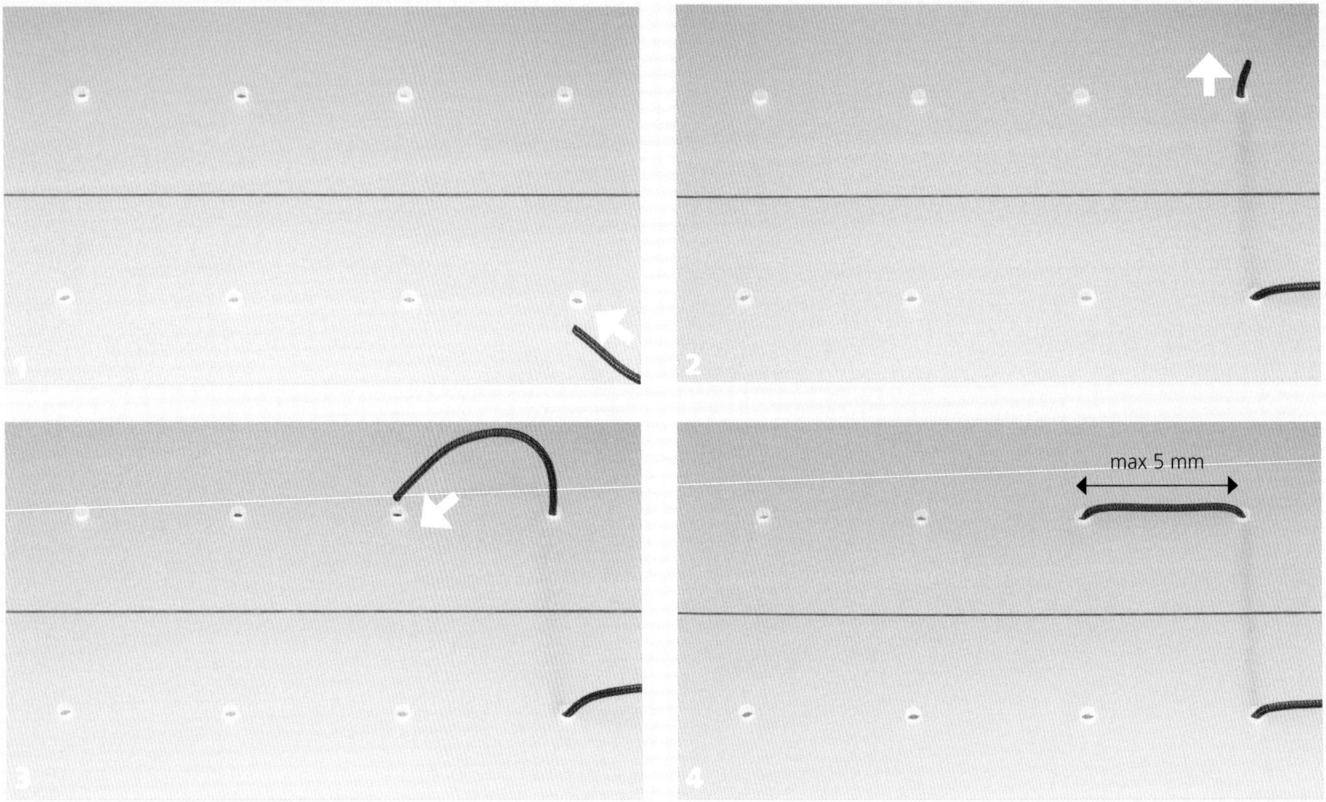

1 The first step is to pierce the mobilized flap from the outside. **2** The thread penetrates the second flap from the inside. **3** The suture is pierced again on the same side from the outside in a line parallel to the wound gap. **4** The distance should not be greater than 5 mm; otherwise, the soft tissues may gather unintentionally.

Schematic representation

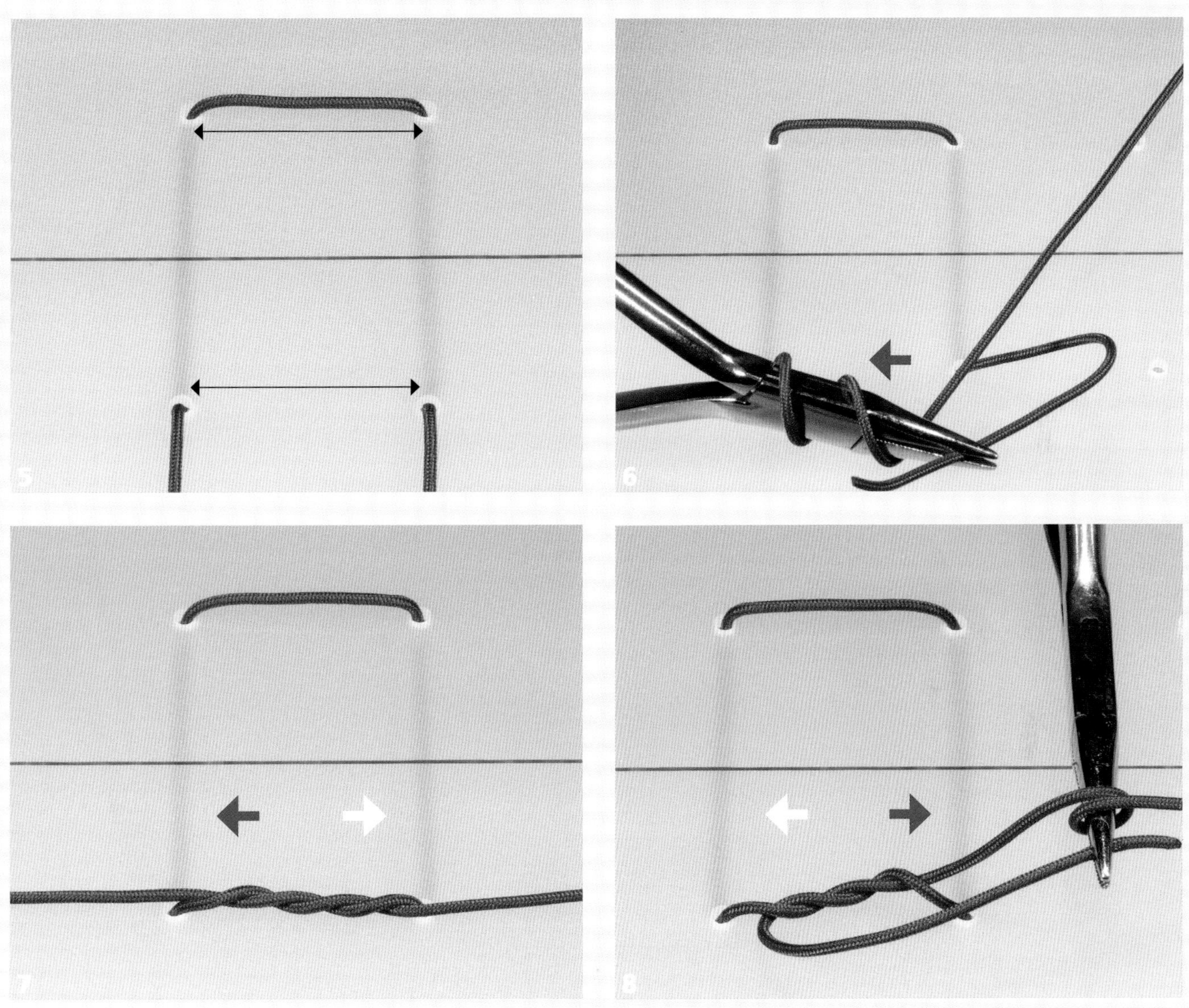

5 Keeping the same distance on both sides, the thread is pierced through the mobile flap to the outside. **6** The knot is made in the same way as with the single button suture. The long end is looped twice around the needle holder. The short end is grasped with the needle holder and pulled through. **7** The knot is tightened and should assume a stable position. It lies straight and shows a spiral pattern. **8** Another knot is made in the opposite direction with a throw.

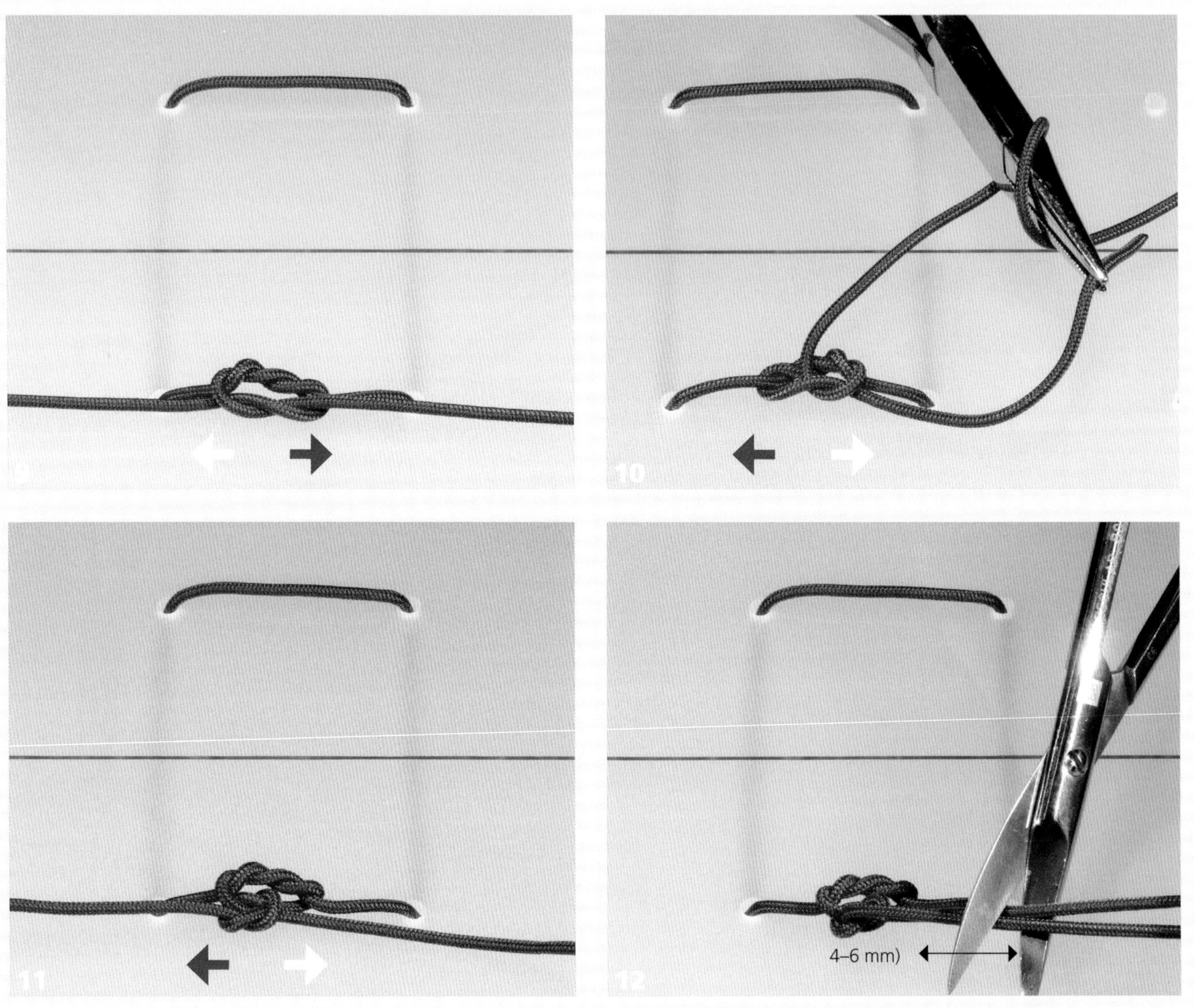

9 The knot is tightened again. Now it can no longer open. **10** Another safety knot with a throw in the same direction as the first knot is made. **11** The third knot is fixed. **12** The knot is shortened with scissors to a thread length of 4 to 6 mm.

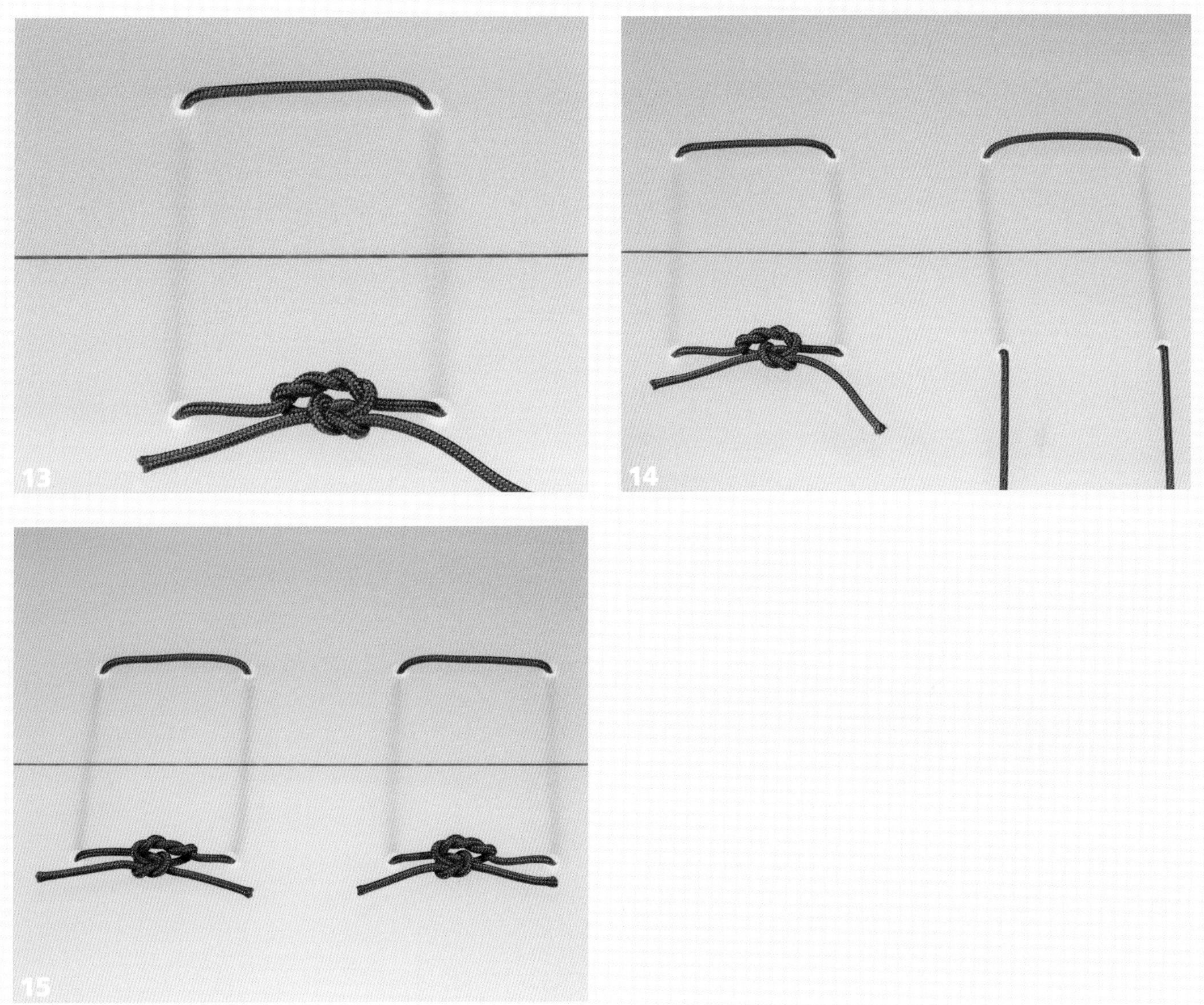

13 Finished horizontal mattress suture. **14** Second horizontal mattress suture before knot formation. **15** Overview of two adjacent horizontal mattress sutures.

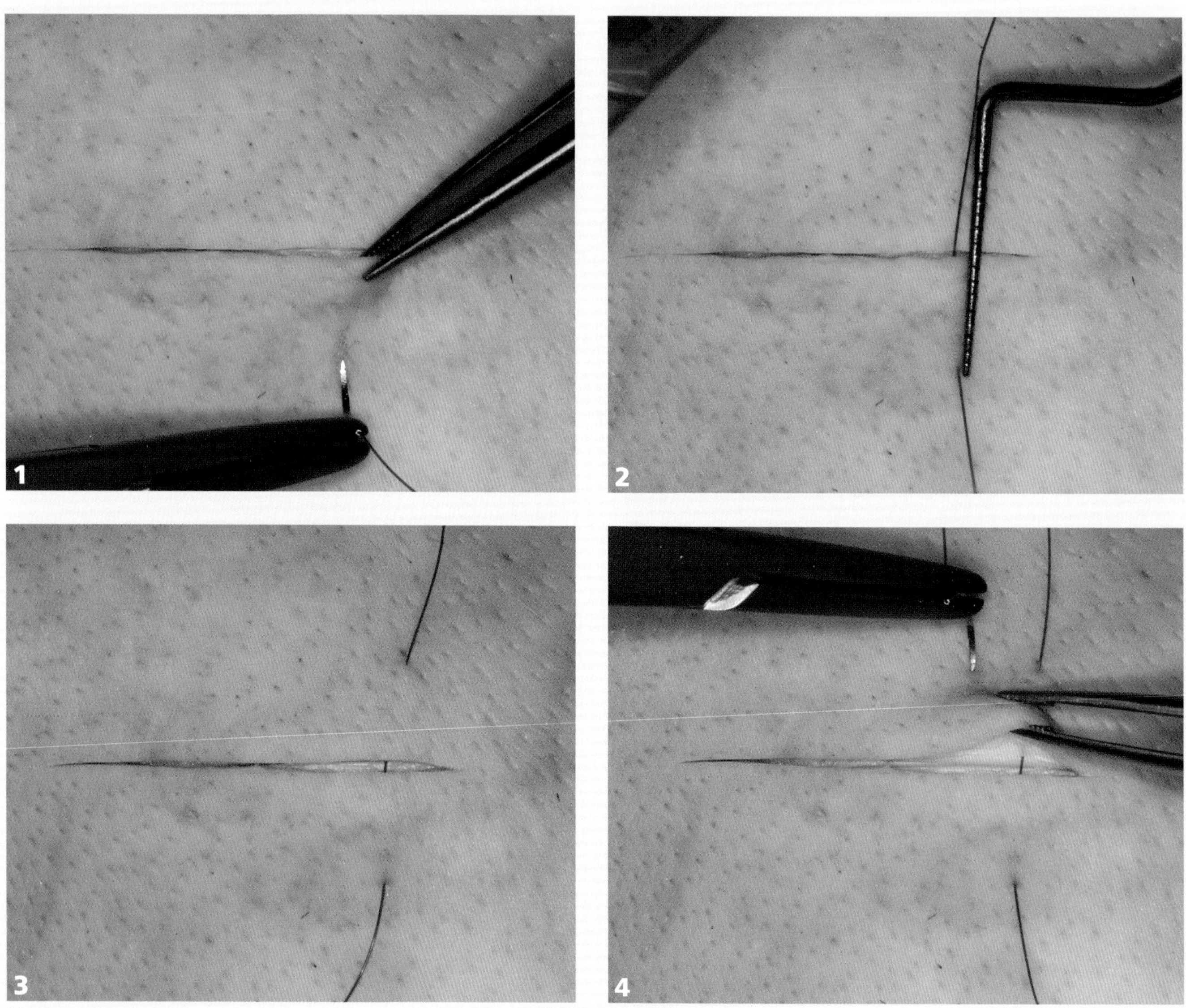

1 The first step is to pierce the mobilized flap from the outside. **2** Ensure sufficient distance to the wound edges (approximately 3 to 5 mm). **3** The suture penetrates the second flap from the inside. **4** The suture is pierced again from the outside on the same side on a line parallel to the wound gap.

Representation on the animal model

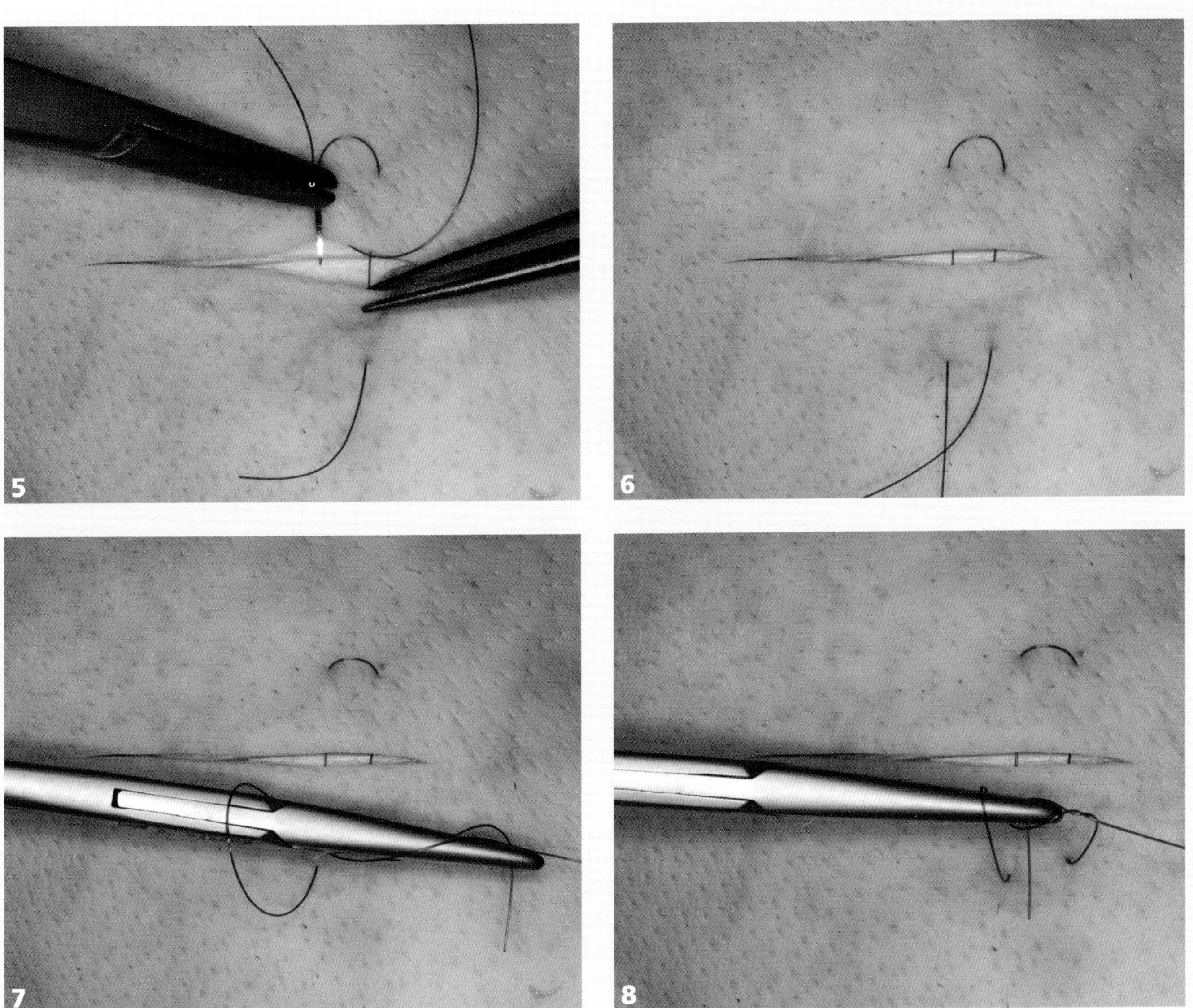

5 Now the thread catches the loop as it exits the tissue and thus fixes itself after being pulled tight through the loop turned by 180 degrees. **6** The seam is continued in this way. The consistent distance between the individual sutures, which are perpendicular to the wound edge (4 to 5 mm), is just as important as the distance between the puncture points and the wound edge (3 to 5 mm). **7** The continuous suture can be extended as desired and is limited only by the total length of the thread. **8** The continuous seam is completed with a knot in the same way as for the single button suture. The long end is looped twice around the needle holder. In this case, the short end is the last thread perpendicular to the wound edge and is grasped with the needle holder.

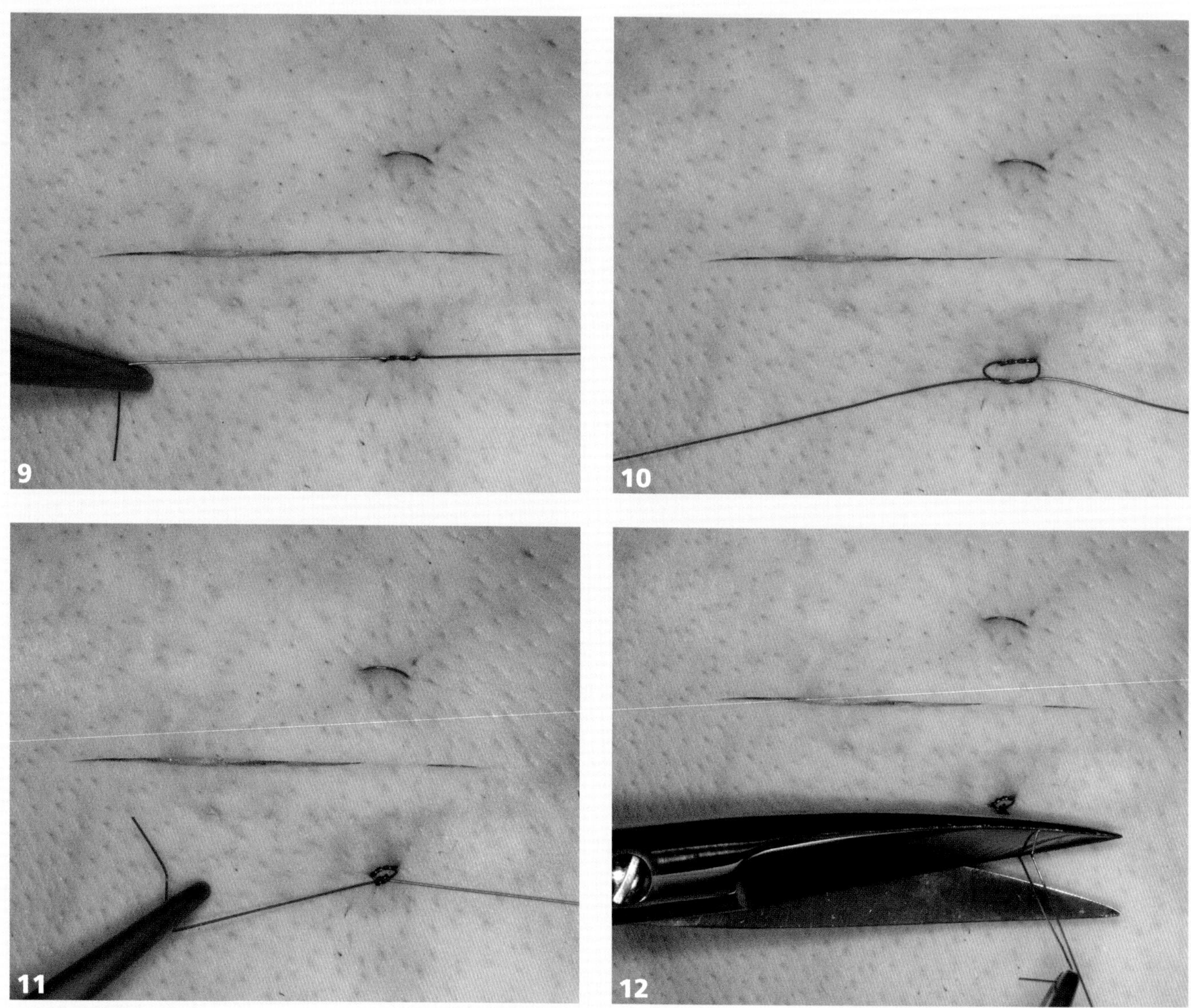

9 The knot lies straight and shows a spiral pattern. **10** The second knot takes place in the opposite direction with a throw. The knot is tightened again. It is now guaranteed that it can no longer open. **11** The third knot follows with a throw in the same direction as the first. **12** The ends of the thread are cut together to a length of approximately 4 to 6 mm.

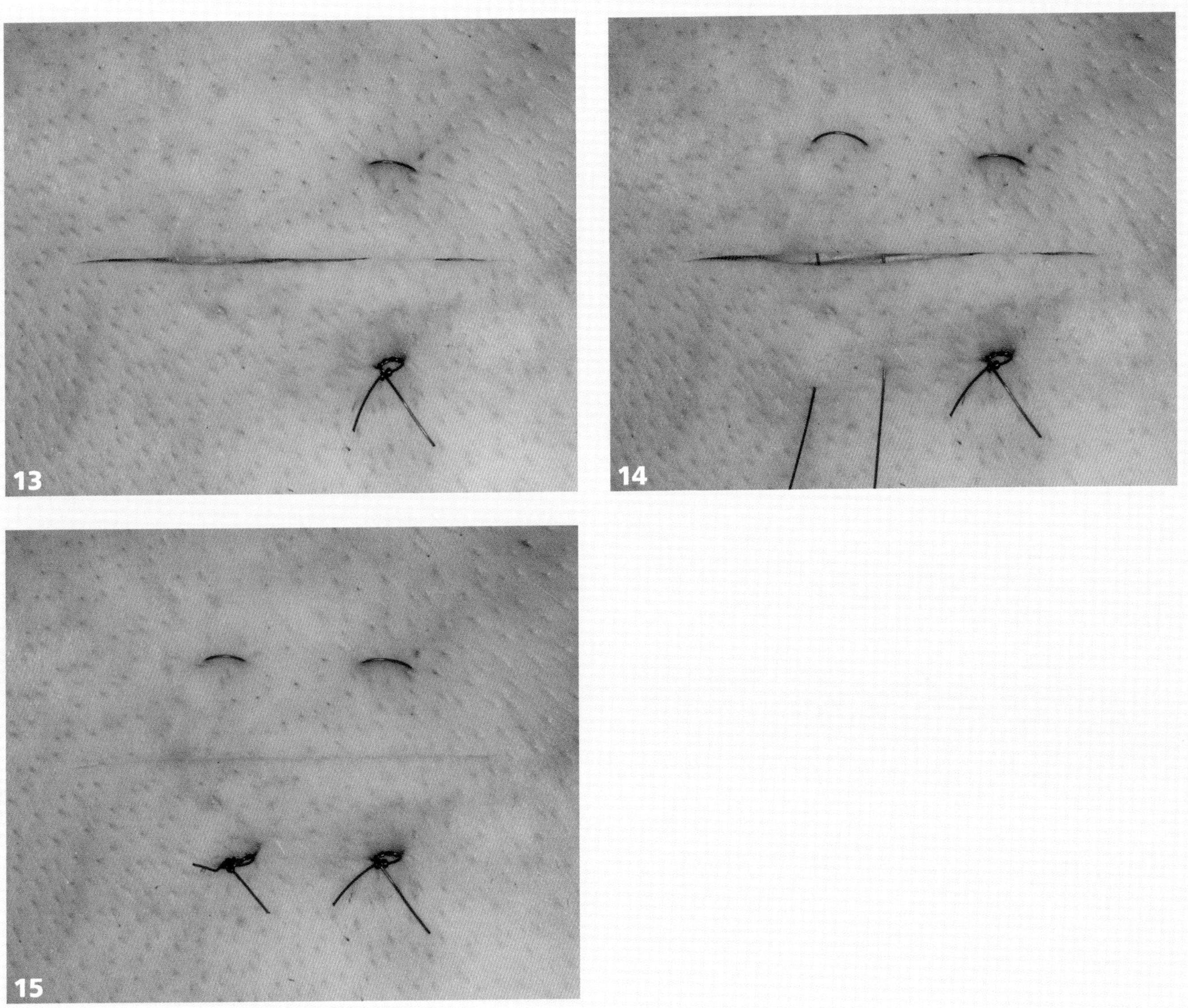

13 The finished horizontal mattress suture shows good adaptation of the wound edges. **14** Second horizontal mattress suture before knot formation. **15** Overview of two adjacent horizontal mattress sutures.

4.2.2 Vertical mattress suture

Indications for mattress sutures:

- Suitable for relieving tension in flaps
- Active positioning of the flap and wound edges
- Used in extractions and periodontal and implant surgery
- Important for coverage after augmentation
- Important for the creation of primary wound closure following, among other things, augmentation procedures

Indication for vertical mattress sutures:

- Used in cases of limited horizontal space (eg, interdentally)

White arrow: Beginning of thread
Gray arrow: End of thread

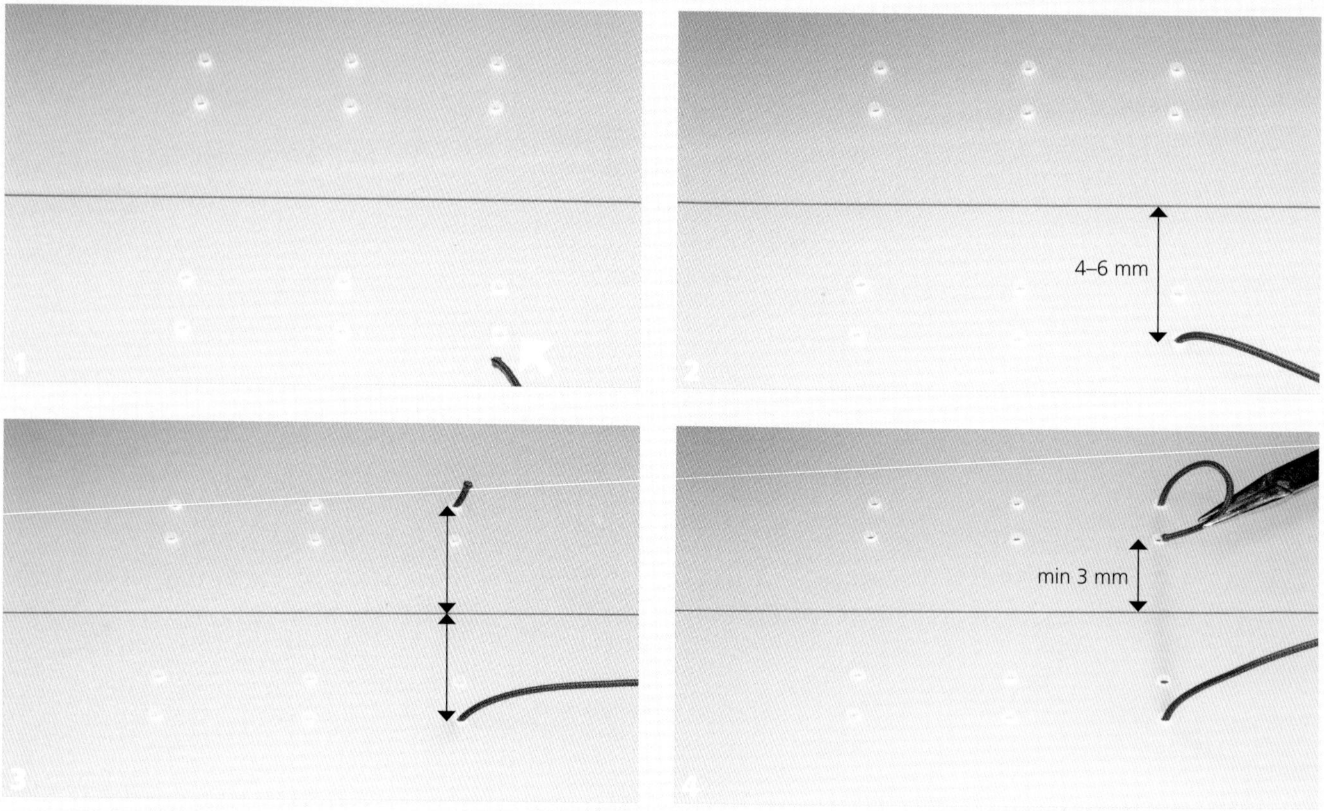

1 The first step is to pierce the mobilized flap from the outside ... **2** ... at a sufficient distance from the wound gap. **3** The suture penetrates the second flap coming from the inside, also at a sufficient distance from the wound gap. **4** The suture is penetrates again on the same side from the outside in a line perpendicular to the wound gap. A minimum distance of 3 mm from the wound gap must be maintained.

Schematic representation

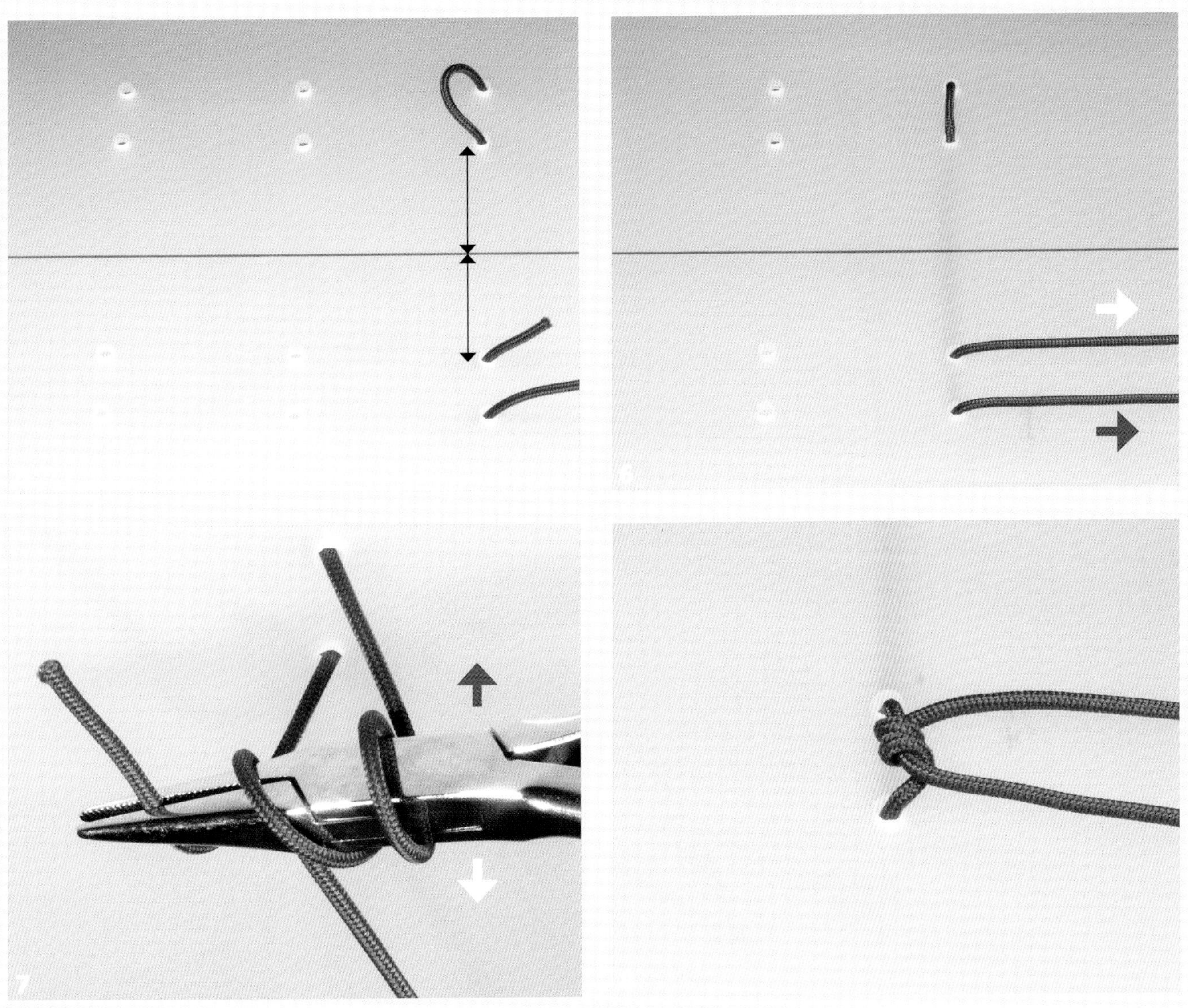

5 Keeping the same distance on both sides, the thread is pierced through the mobile flap to the outside. **6** Moderate traction is used to check whether the wound edges can be adapted by this measure. **7** The knot is tied in the same way as for the single button suture. The long end is looped twice around the needle holder. The short end is grasped with the needle holder and pulled through. **8** The knot is tightened and should assume a stable position. It lies straight and shows a spiral pattern.

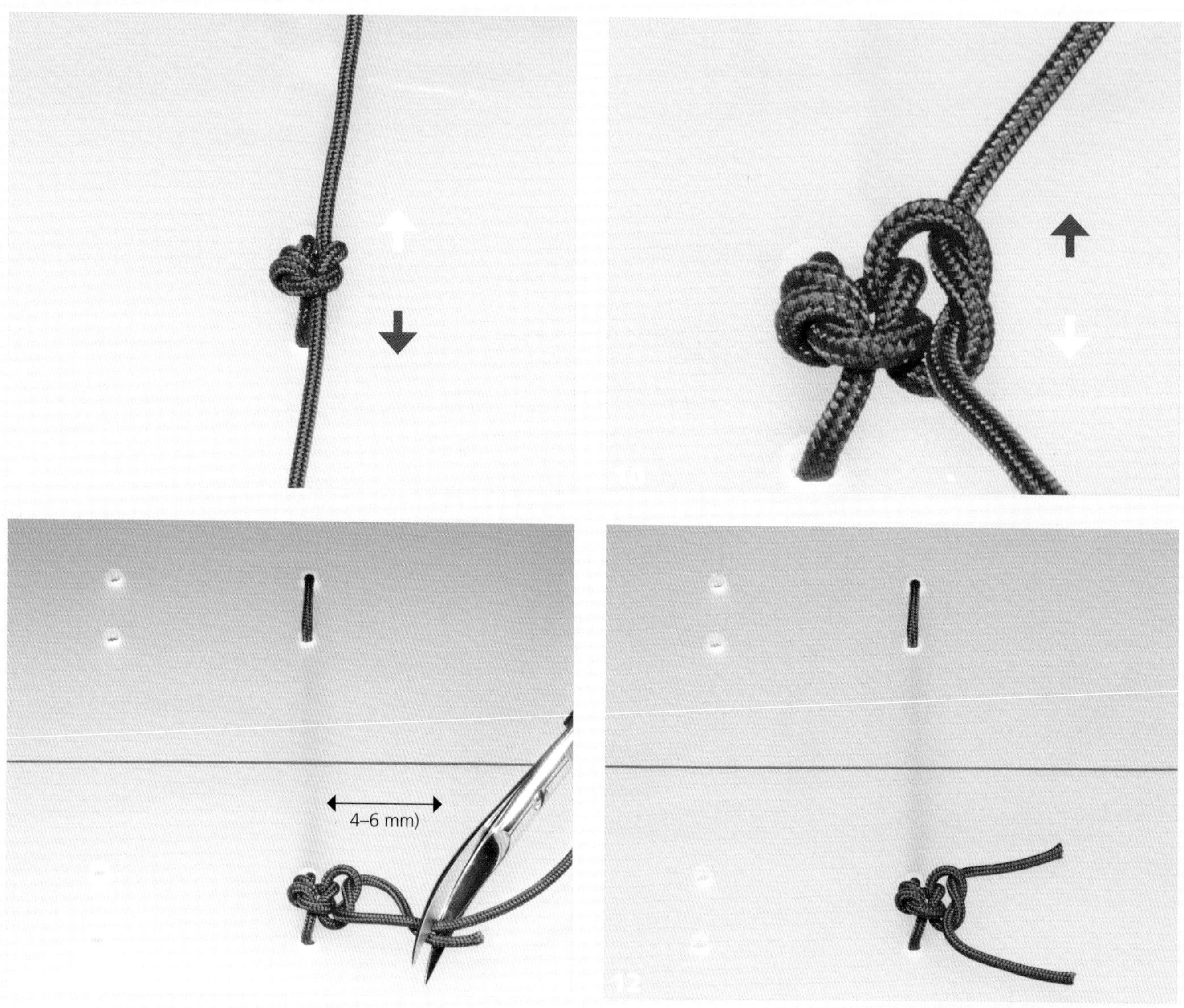

9 Another knot is made in the opposite direction with a throw. **10** Another safety knot is made with a throw in the same direction as the first knot. **11** Using the scissors, the knot is cut to a thread length of 4 to 6 mm. **12** Finished vertical mattress suture; if this suture is used interdentally, the papillae tips will stand up, and an additional single button suture will be necessary.

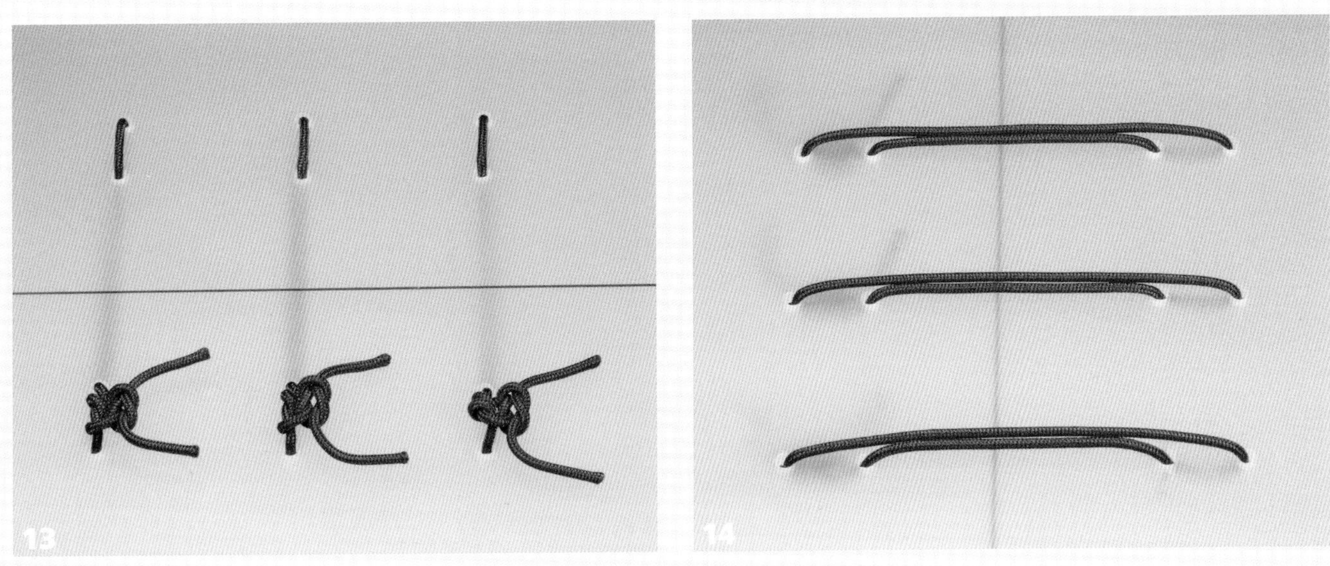

13 Three vertical mattress suture arranged parallel to each other. **14** Overview of vertical mattress sutures "from below" (tissue side).

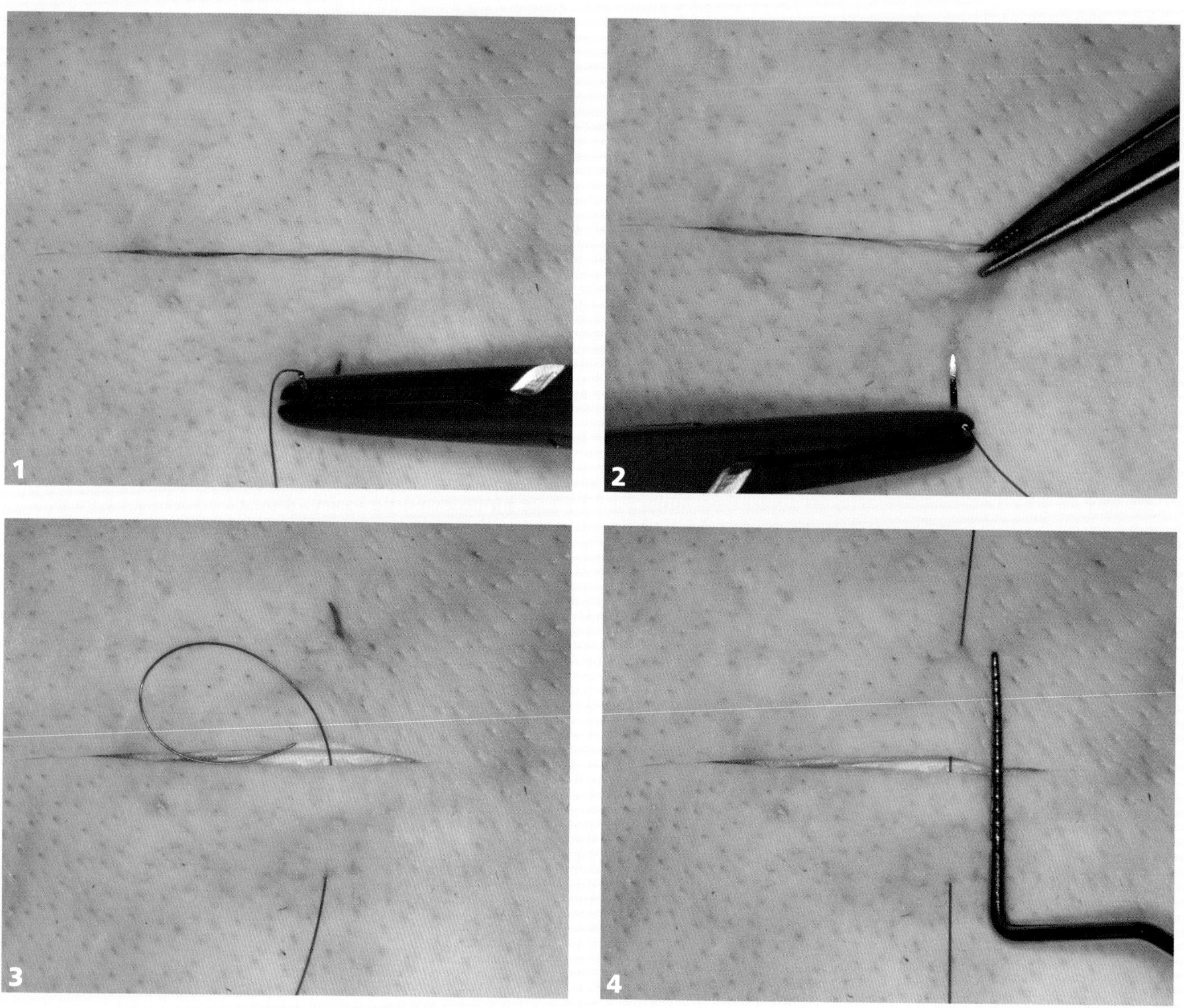

1 The flap is penetrated from the outside to the inside with sufficient distance from the wound edge. **2** The needle tip is picked up after the tissue has been penetrated. **3** The needle penetrates the second flap from the inside to the outside, also with sufficient distance from the wound margin. **4** The periodontal probe shows the distances to the wound margin.

Representation on the animal model

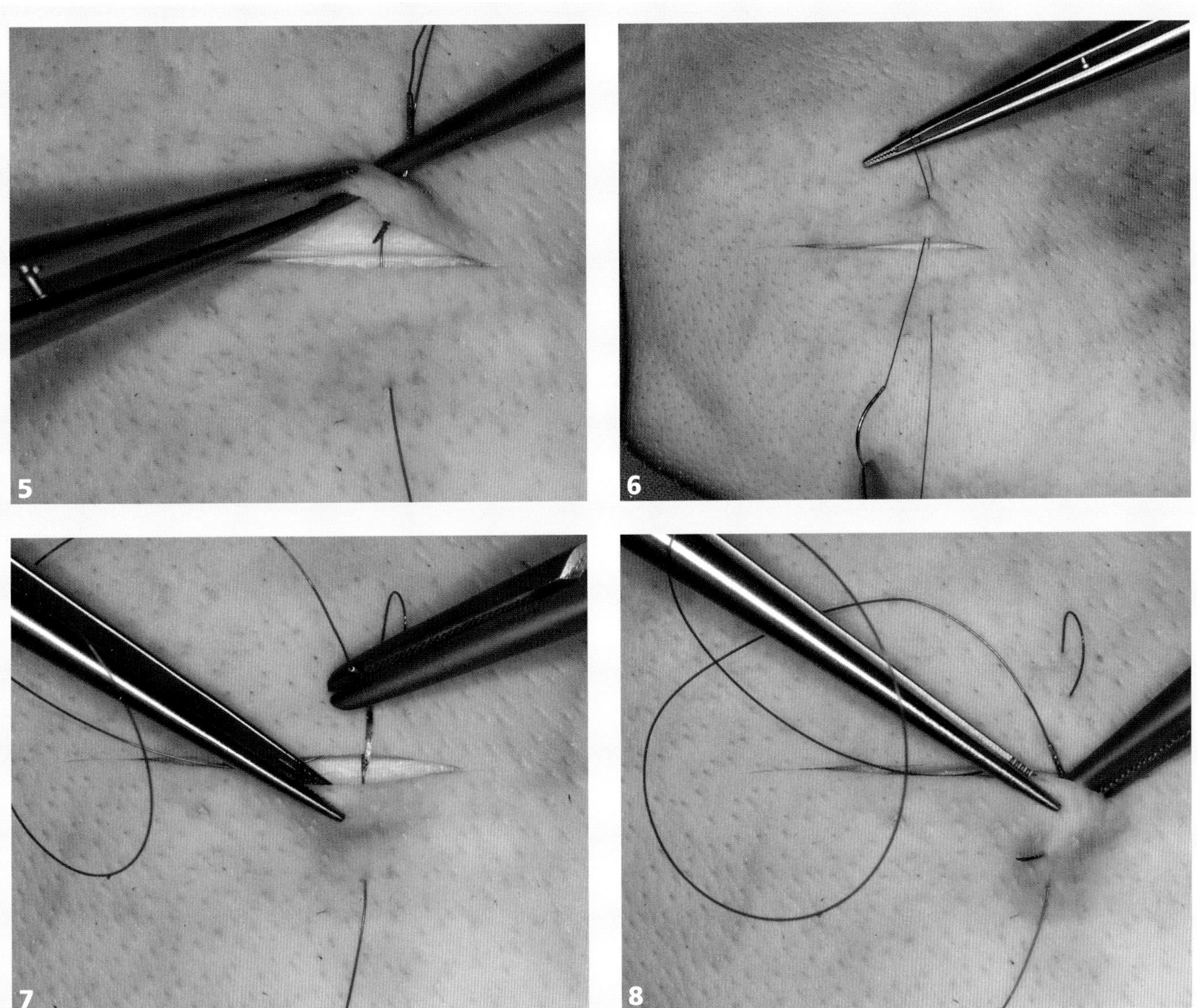

5 The suture is pierced again from the outside on the same side in a line perpendicular to the wound gap. A minimum distance of 3 mm from the wound gap must be maintained. **6** The suture is pulled back and deflected over an instrument (here: forceps) to protect the tissue. **7** In the usual manner, the flap end is held with the forceps to allow penetration with the needle. **8** Keeping the same distance on both sides, the thread is pierced through the mobile flap to the outside.

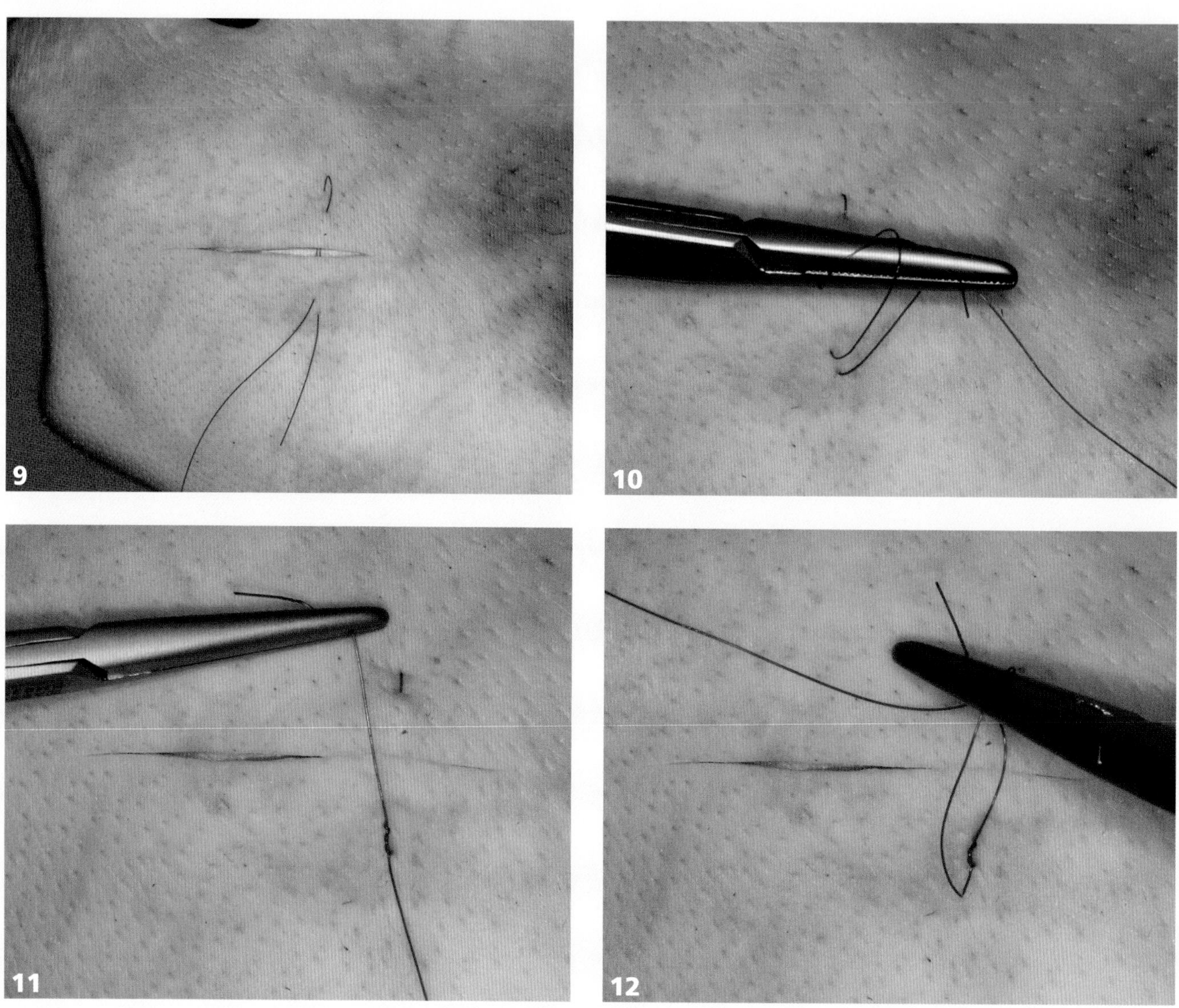

9 The thread is in position for knot tying. **10** The knot is tied in the same way as with the single button suture. The long end is looped twice around the needle holder. The short end is grasped with the needle holder and pulled through. **11** The knot is pulled tight and should assume a stable position. It lies straight and shows a spiral pattern. **12** Another knot is made in the opposite direction with a throw.

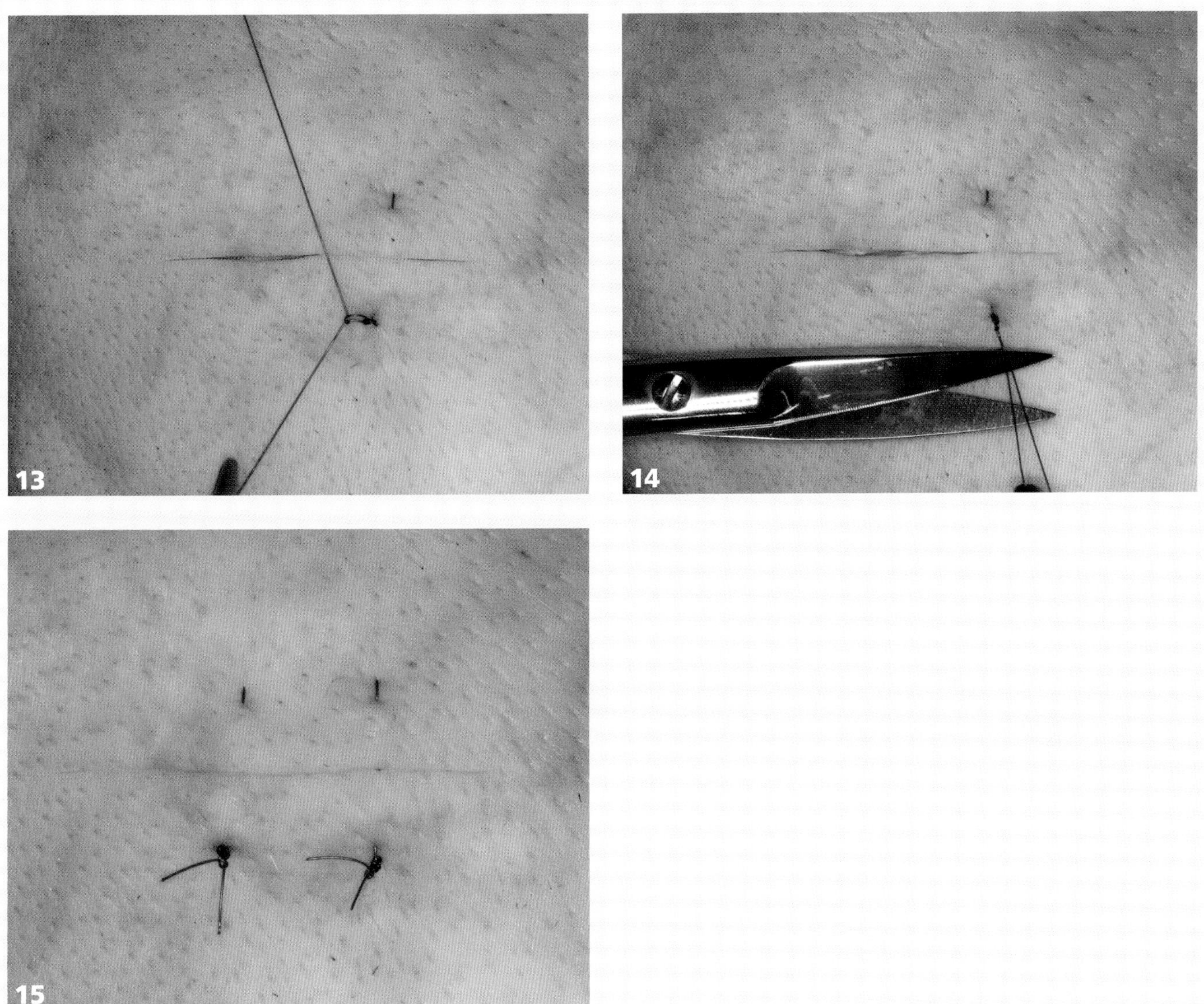

13 Another safety knot is made with a throw in the same direction as the first knot. **14** The knot is cut with scissors to a thread length of 4 to 6 mm. **15** Two vertical mattress sutures arranged parallel to each other in situ.

4.2.3 Cross mattress suture

Indications for mattress sutures:

- Suitable for relieving tension in flaps
- Active positioning of the flap and wound edges
- Used in extractions and periodontal and implant surgery
- Important for coverage after augmentation
- Important for the creation of primary wound closure following, among other things, augmentation procedures

Indications for cross mattress sutures:

- Used in extractions to stabilize the blood coagulum and the wound edges
- In the case of inhomogeneous alveolar ridge anatomy, used to achieve stable adaptation of the wound margins

White arrow: Beginning of thread
Gray arrow: End of thread

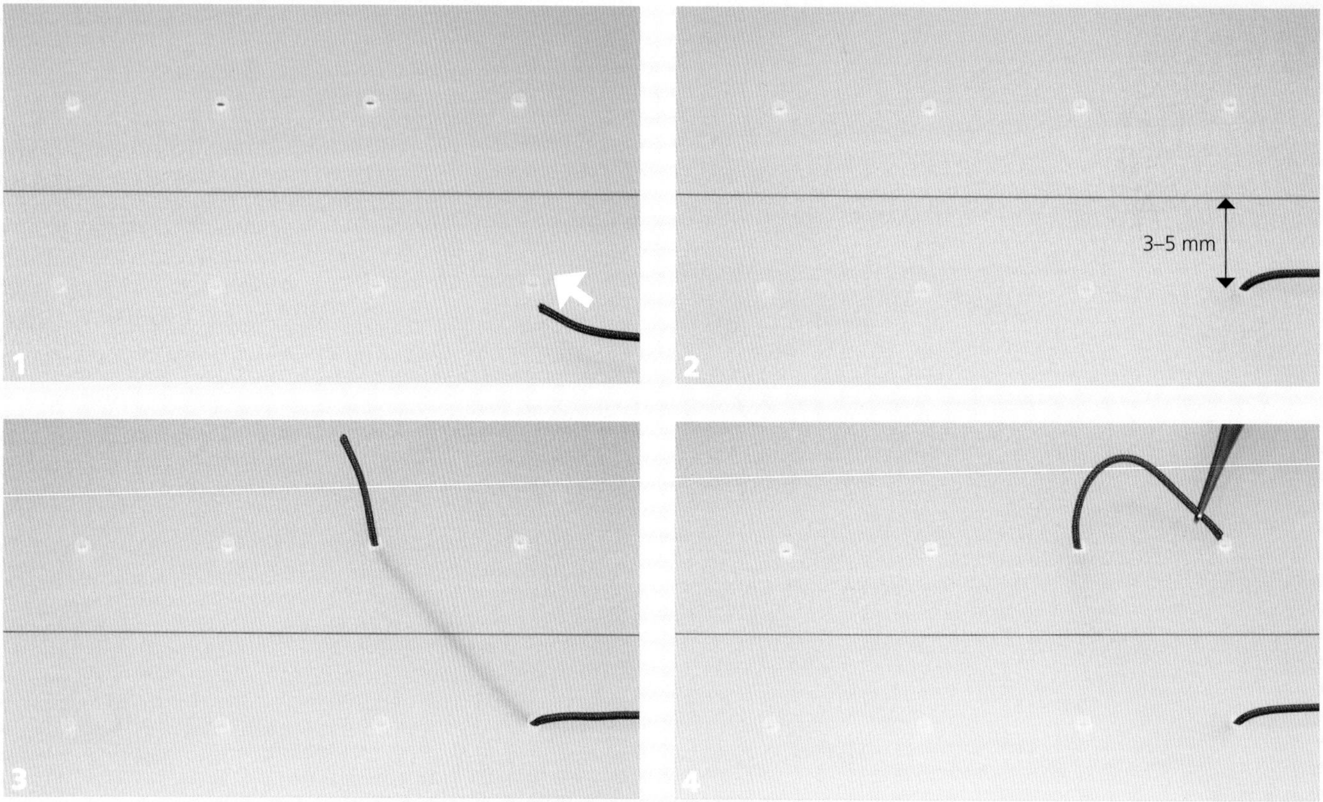

1 The first step is to pierce the mobilized flap from the outside ... **2** ... at a sufficient distance from the wound gap. **3** The suture penetrates the second flap from the inside to the outside, but not perpendicular to the wound gap. **4** The suture is penetrates again on the same side from the outside in a line parallel to the wound gap, to the right or in the direction of the original penetration. A distance of 3 to 5 mm from the wound gap must be maintained.

Schematic representation

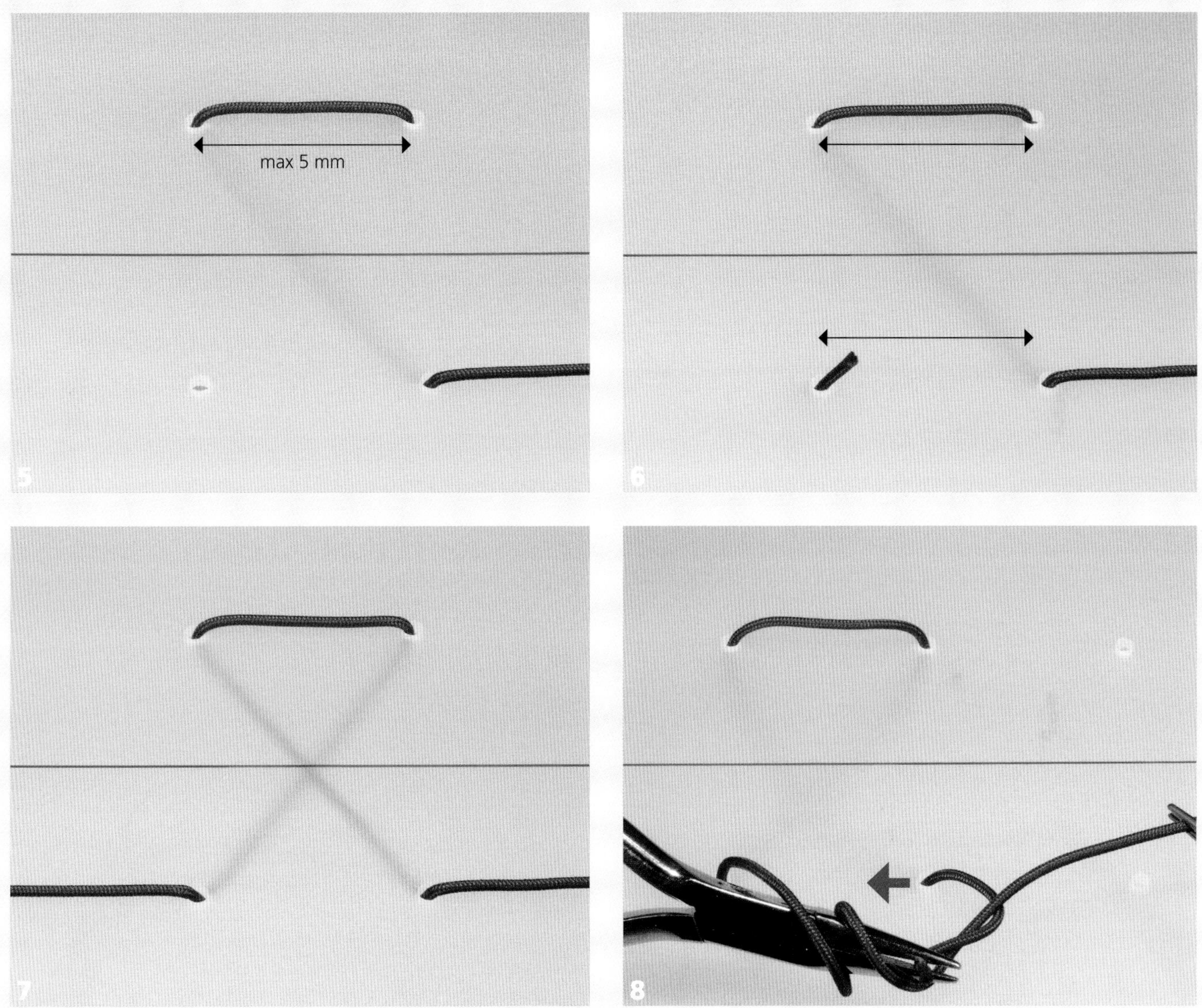

5 The distance between the puncture points on one side of the wound gap should not be greater than 5 mm; otherwise, the soft tissues may gather unintentionally. **6** While maintaining the same distance on both sides, the suture is pierced outward through the mobile flap. **7** The crossing of the suture at the level of the wound gap is clearly visible. **8** The knot is tied in the same way as for the single button suture. The long end is looped twice around the needle holder. The short end is grasped with the needle holder and pulled through.

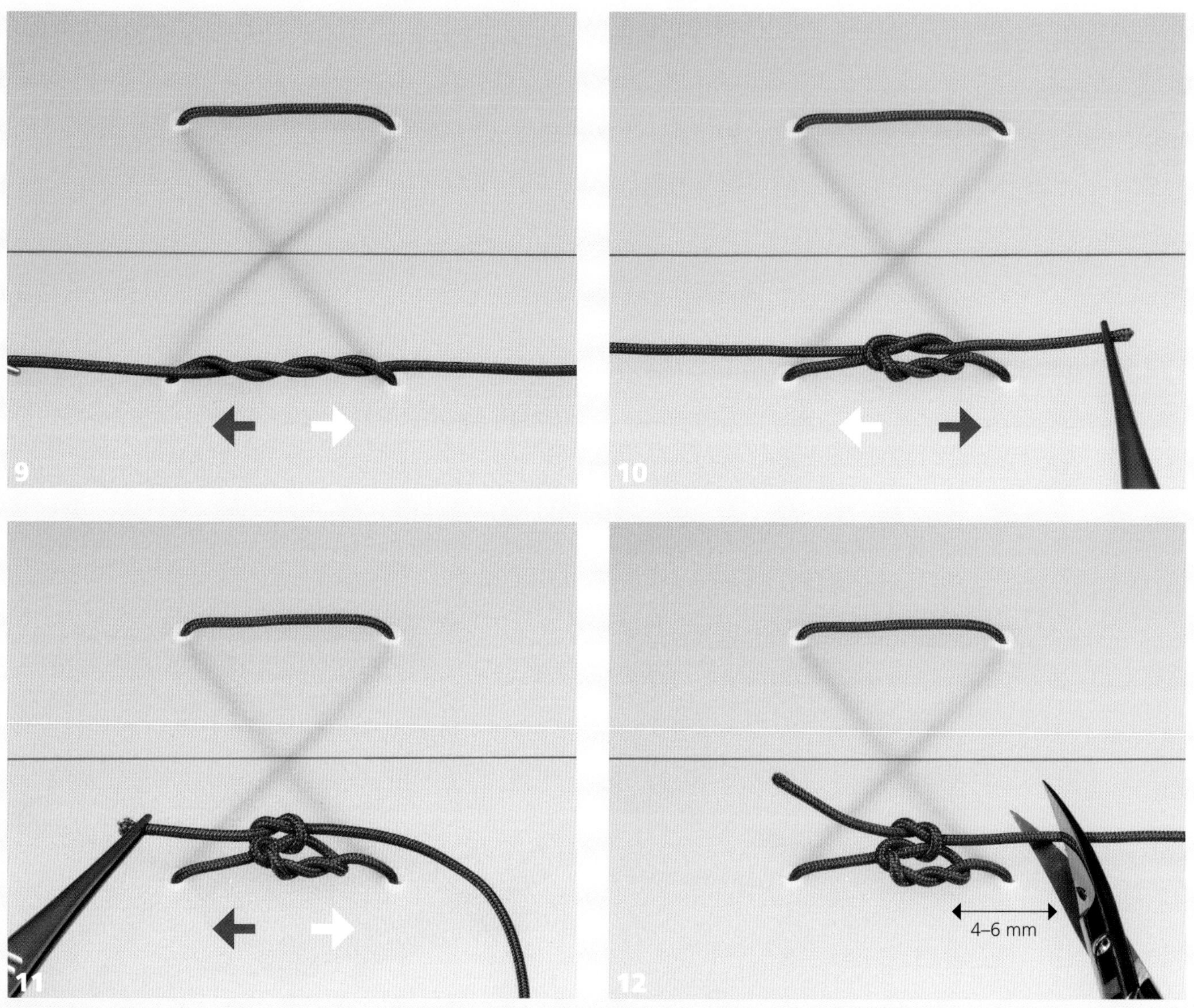

9 The knot is tightened and should assume a stable position. It lies straight and shows a spiral pattern. **10** Another knot is made in the opposite direction with a throw. **11** Another safety knot is made with a throw in the same direction as the first knot. **12** The knot is cut to a thread length of 4 to 6 mm with the scissors.

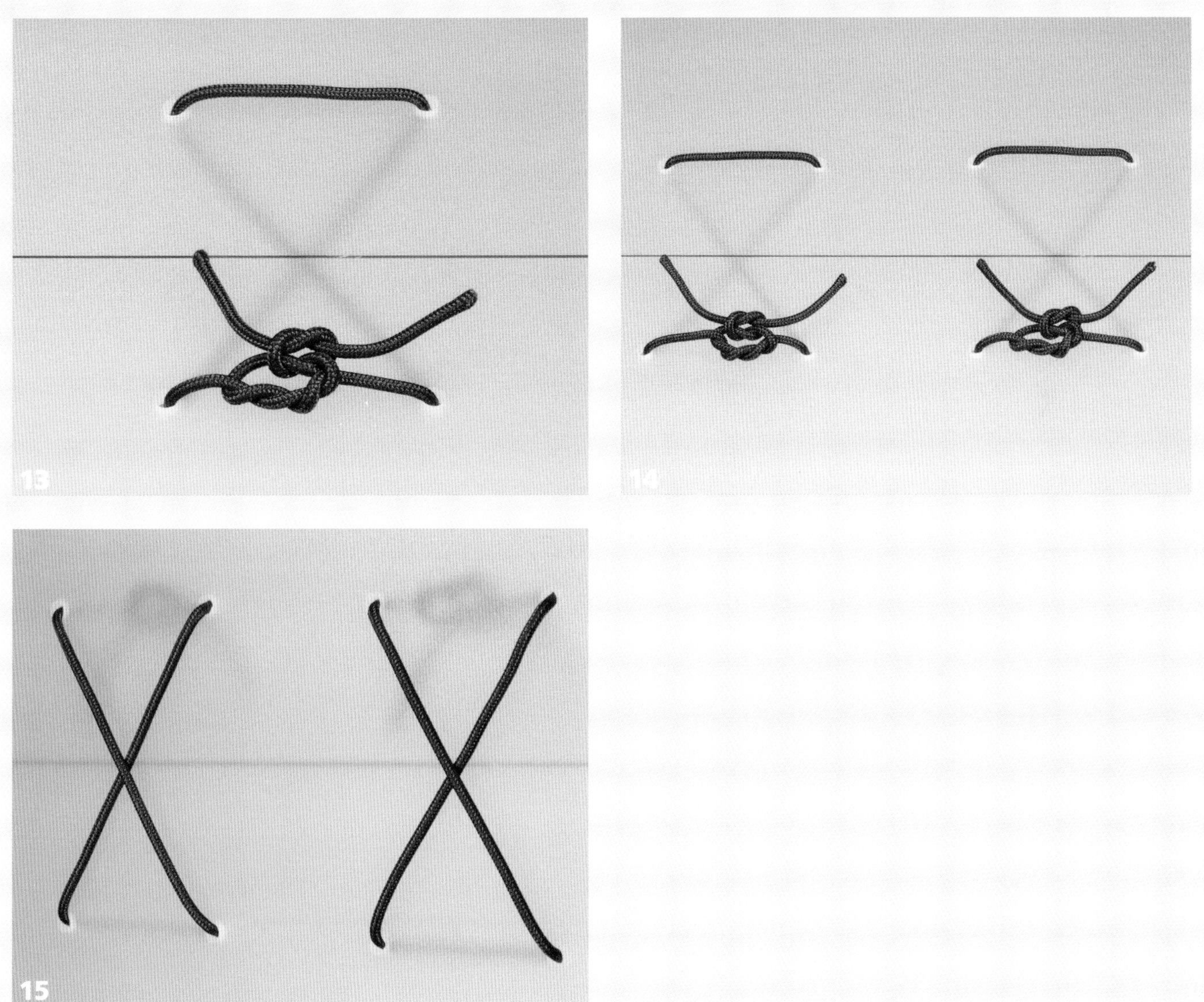

13 Finished cross mattress suture. **14** Two vertical mattress sutures arranged parallel to each other. **15** Overview of cross mattress sutures "from below" (tissue side).

No representation on the animal specimen, where the cross mattress suture is visually indistinguishable from the horizontal mattress suture.

4.3 Laurell suture

4.3.1 Horizontal Laurell suture

Indications for Laurell sutures:

- Suitable for relieving tension in flaps
- Active positioning of the flap and wound edges
- Used in extractions and periodontal and implant surgery
- Helps with coverage after augmentation procedures
- Helps in the creation of primary wound closure

Note: Also referred to as the Laurell-Gottlow suture; combination of mattress and single button sutures.

- Advantage: Saves time.
- Disadvantages: If part of the thread comes loose, the entire suture comes undone; the position of the single button suture depends on the position of the mattress suture.

White arrow: Beginning of thread
Gray arrow: End of thread

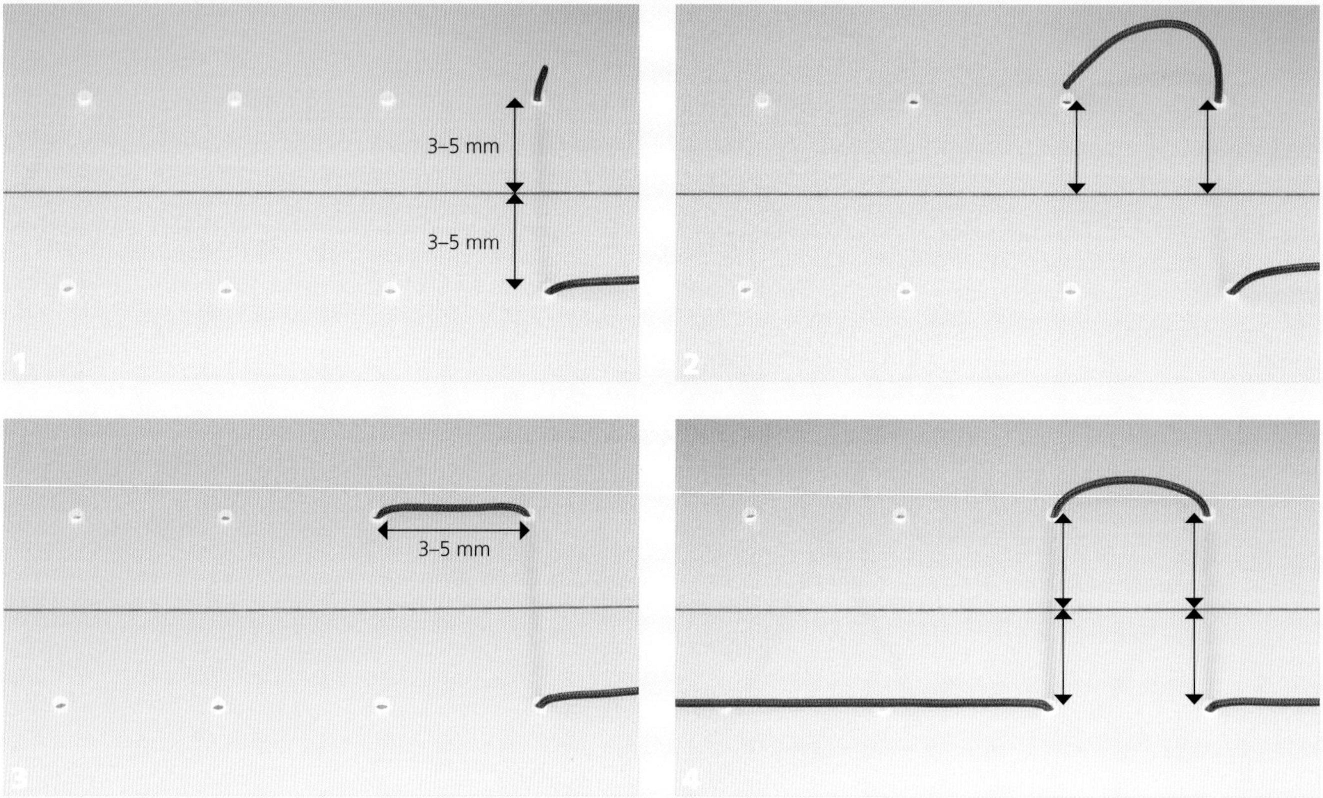

3–5 mm
3–5 mm

3–5 mm

1 The mobilized flap is pierced from the outside, and then the needle penetrates the second flap at the same distance from the incision line from the inside. **2** The needle is then turned, and the second flap is penetrated again at the same distance from the incision line. The distance between the two puncture sites on the second flap has an influence on the wound margins. **3** The greater the distance between the two puncture sites on the second flap, the greater the protrusion of the wound edges. **4** The mobilized flap is pierced a second time, maintaining the same distance from the incision line from the inside to the outside. The mattress suture is completed. The two thread ends are carefully tightened until a small loop is formed on the side of the second flap.

Schematic representation

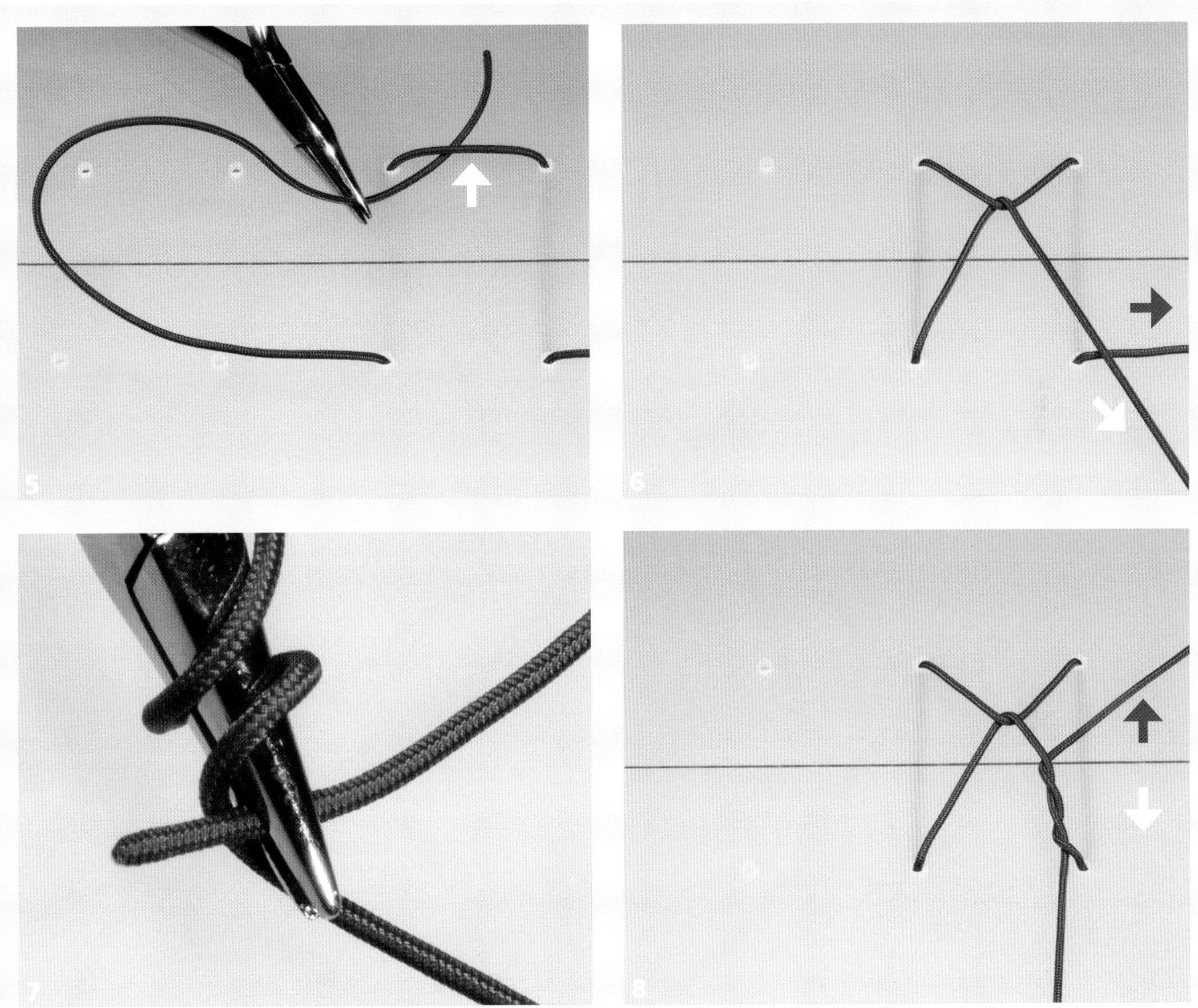

5 Before knotting, the suture is picked up again with the forceps and passed through the loop on the second flap from the incision side. **6** By pulling on both ends of the thread, the flap can be actively positioned, and the wound edges can be set up. **7** Now the knot formation takes place. The long thread end is looped twice around the needle holder, and the short end is grasped with the needle holder. **8** The knot is tightened, showing a spiral pattern and assuming a stable position.

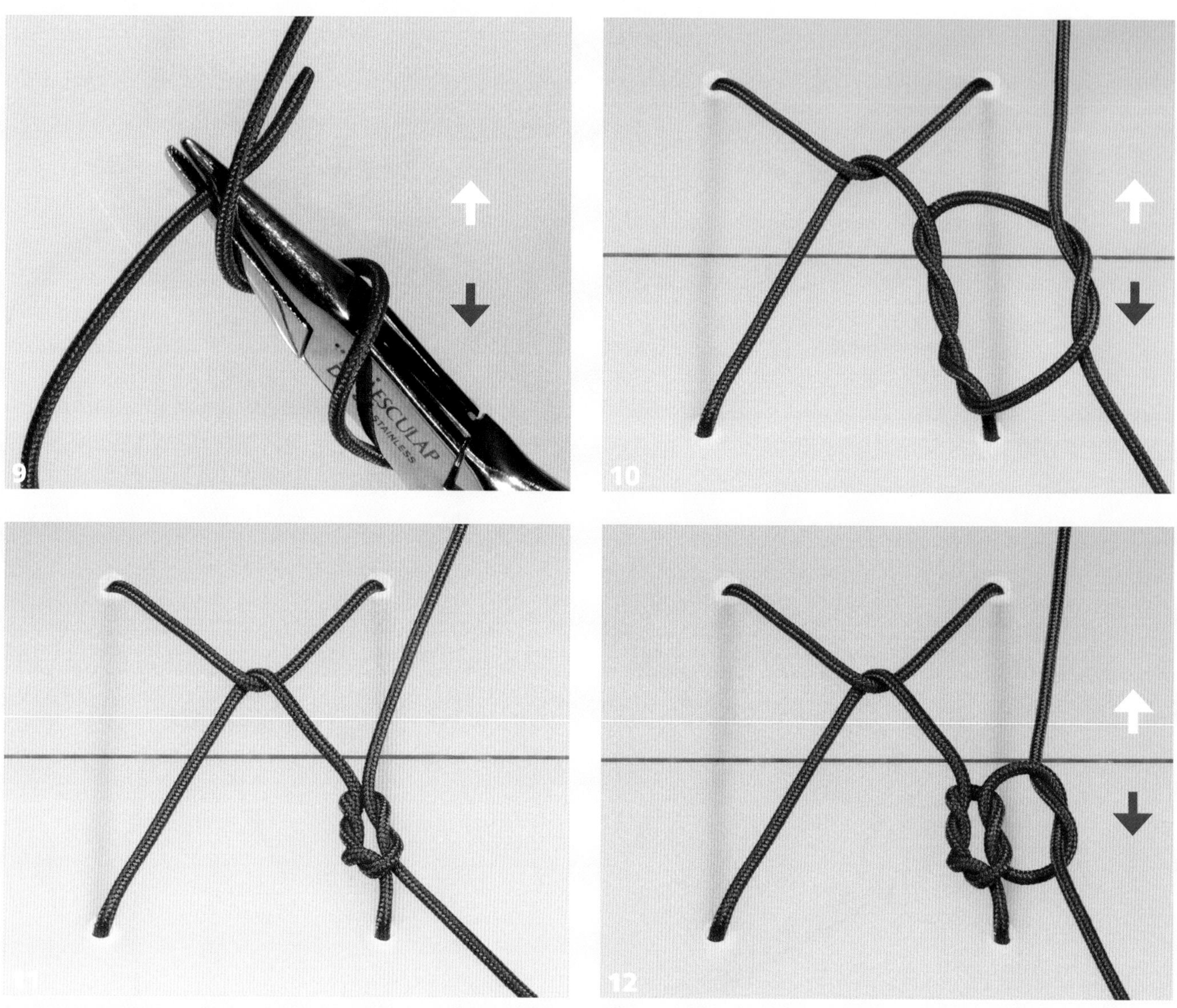

9 The second knot is made in the opposite direction with a throw. **10** The knot is tightened again and is now firmly seated. **11** The knot should be positioned away from the wound margin, preferably on the side of the keratinized gingiva. **12** A third safety knot in the same direction as the first finalizes the surgical knot.

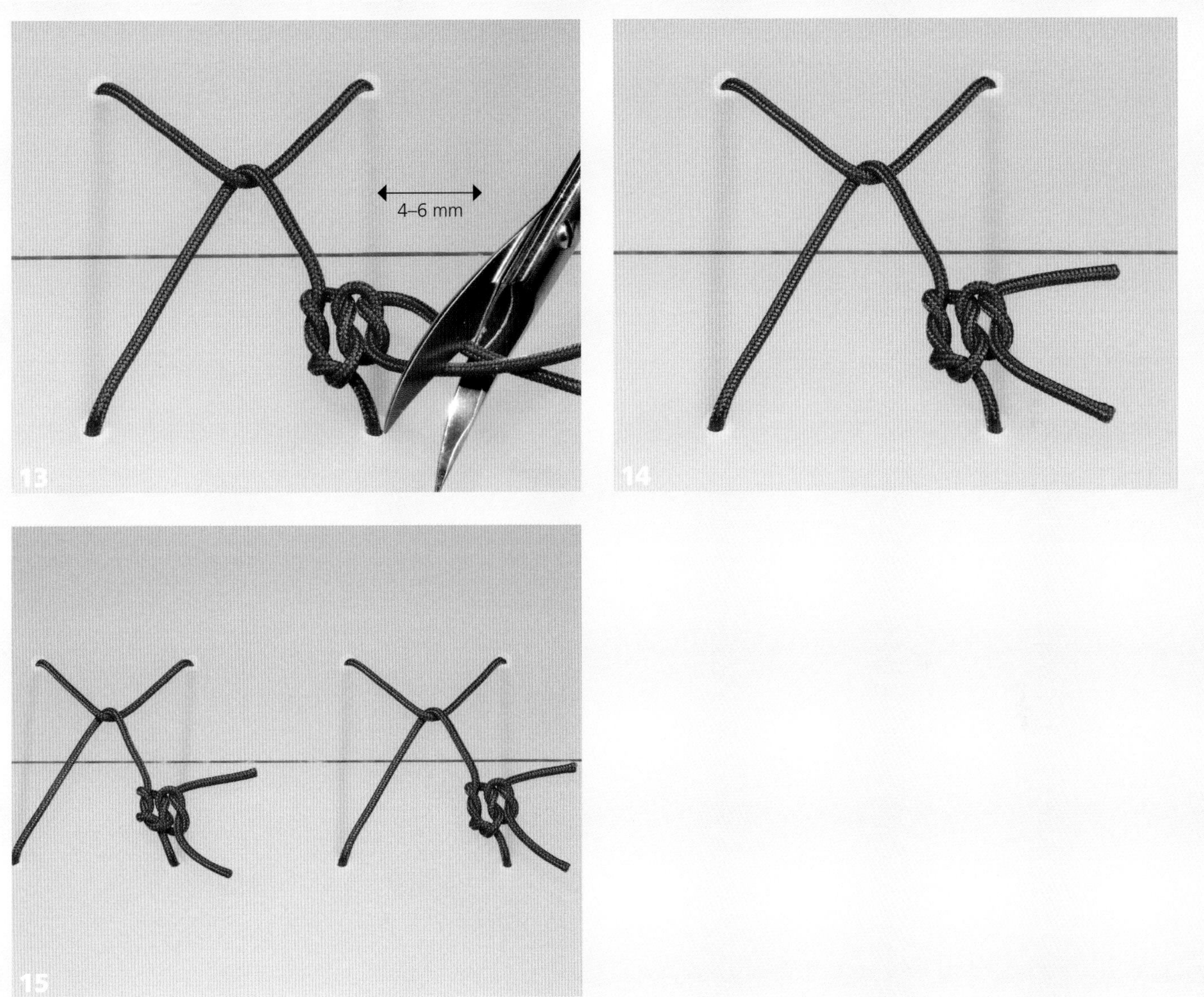

13 The knot is cut to a length of 4 to 6 mm with scissors. **14** A finished horizontal Laurell suture. **15** Overview of two adjacent horizontal Laurell sutures.

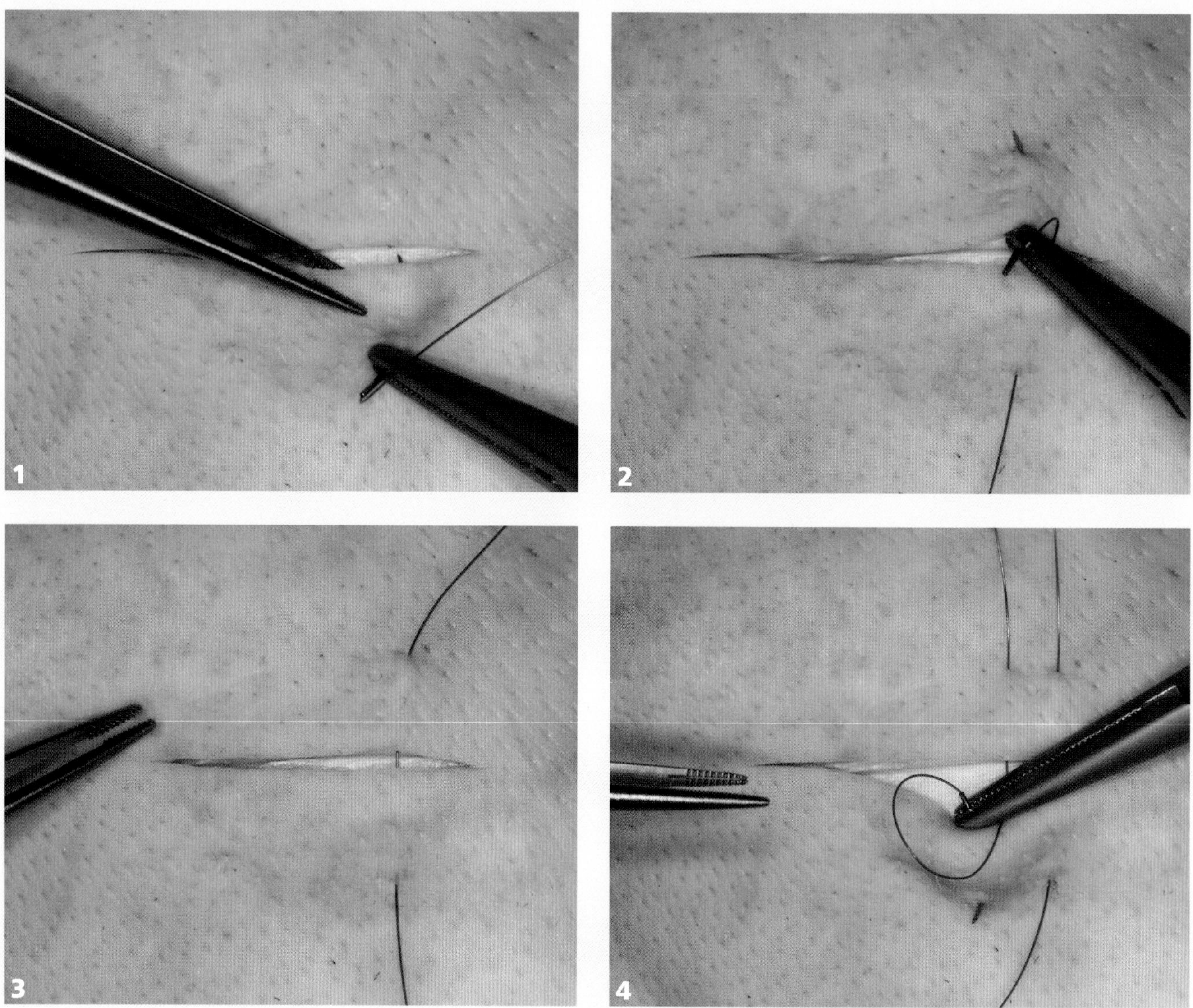

1 In a first step, the mobilized flap is penetrated from the outside to the inside. **2** The suture penetrates the second flap from the inside to the outside. **3** Ensure sufficient distance to the wound edges (3 to 5 mm). **4** After passing the suture on a line parallel to the wound gap on the same side from the outside to the inside, pierce it from the inside outward through the mobile flap while maintaining the same distance on both sides.

Representation on the animal model

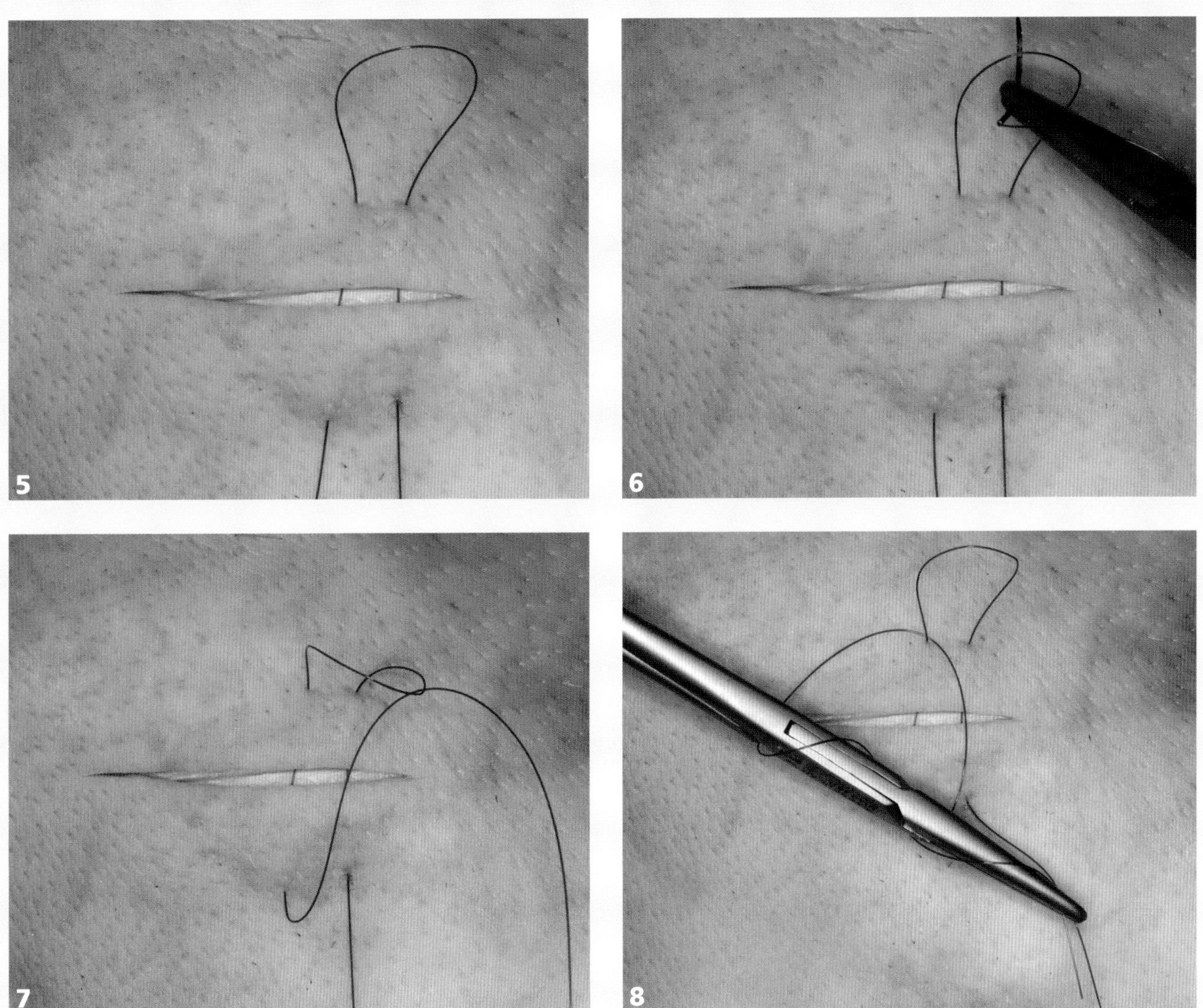

5 The distance between the two puncture points parallel to the wound edge should not be greater than 5 mm; otherwise, undesirable gathering of the soft tissue may occur. The two ends of the thread should be tightened until a loop is formed on the second flap.
6 The suture is then picked up with the forceps and passed through the loop from the incision side. **7** The two ends of the thread are carefully tightened before knot formation. **8** Knot formation is performed in the same way as for single button suturing. The long thread end is looped twice around the needle holder, and the short thread end is grasped with the needle holder.

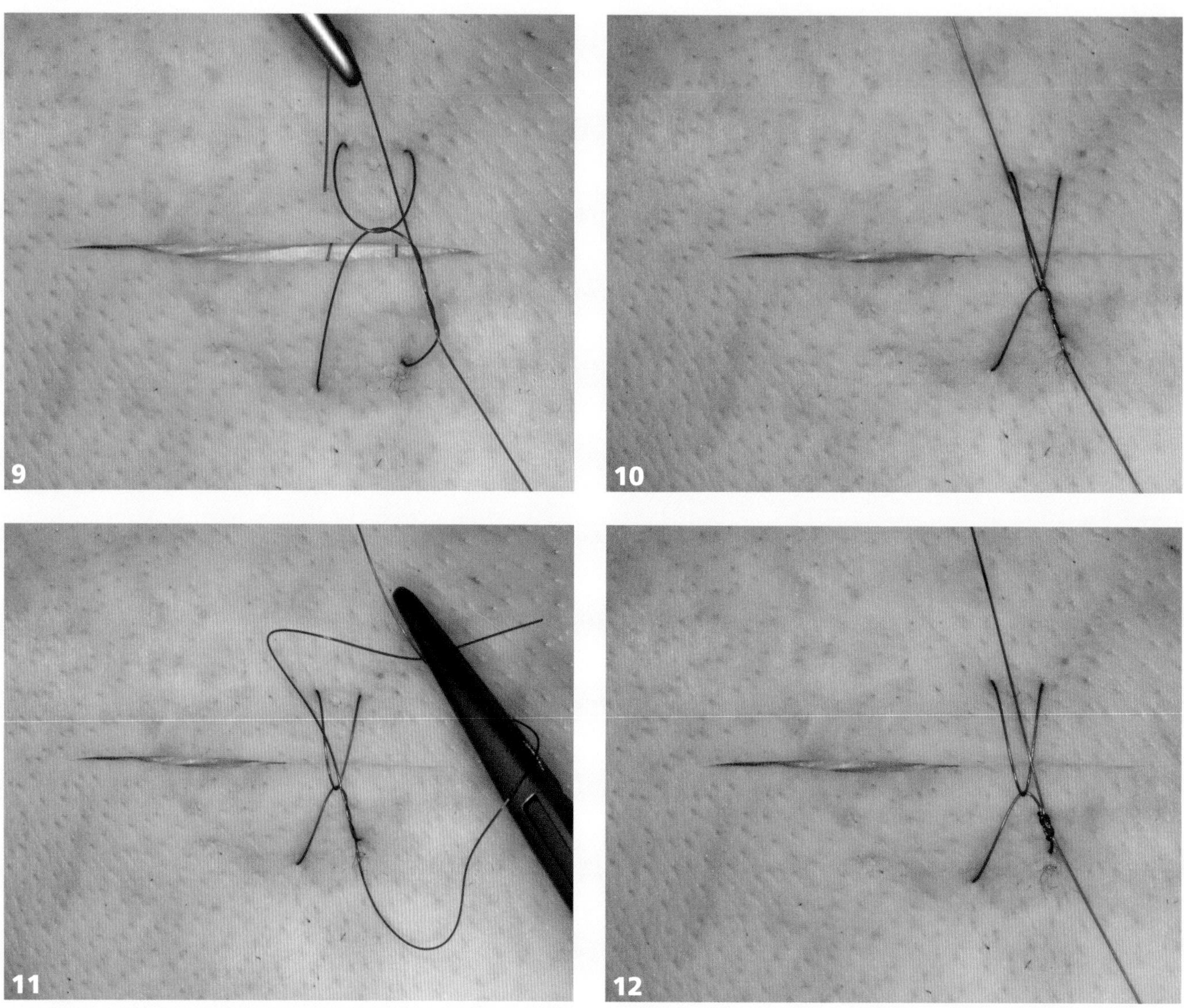

9 The knot is carefully tightened. **10** The knot lies straight and shows a spiral pattern. It should preferably lie on the side of the keratinized gingiva away from the wound margin. **11** The second knot is placed in the opposite direction with a throw. **12** It is now ensured that it can no longer open.

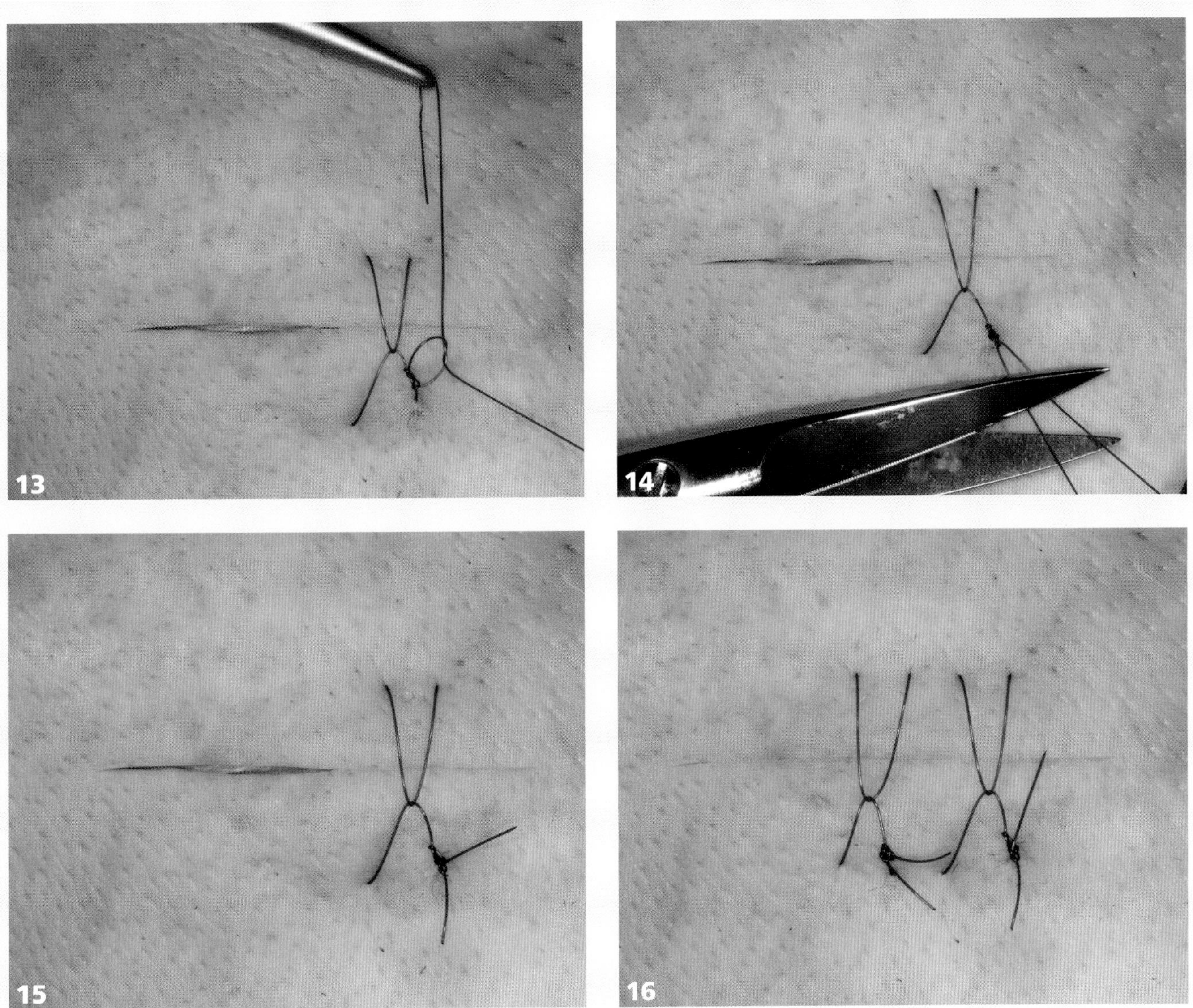

13 A third knot for safety is made in the opposite direction to the first knot. **14** Use scissors to cut the thread ends to a length of 4 to 6 mm. **15** Finished horizontal Laurell suture. **16** Two horizontal Laurell sutures side by side.

4.3.2 Vertical Laurell suture

Indications for Laurell sutures:

- Suitable for relieving tension in flaps
- Active positioning of the flap and wound edges
- Used in extractions and periodontal and implant surgery
- Helps with coverage after augmentation procedures
- Helps in the creation of primary wound closure

Note:

- Also referred to as the Laurell-Gottlow suture; combination of mattress and single button sutures.
- Advantage: Saves time.
- Disadvantages: If part of the thread comes loose, the entire suture comes undone; the position of the single button suture depends on the position of the mattress suture.

White arrow: Beginning of thread
Gray arrow: End of thread

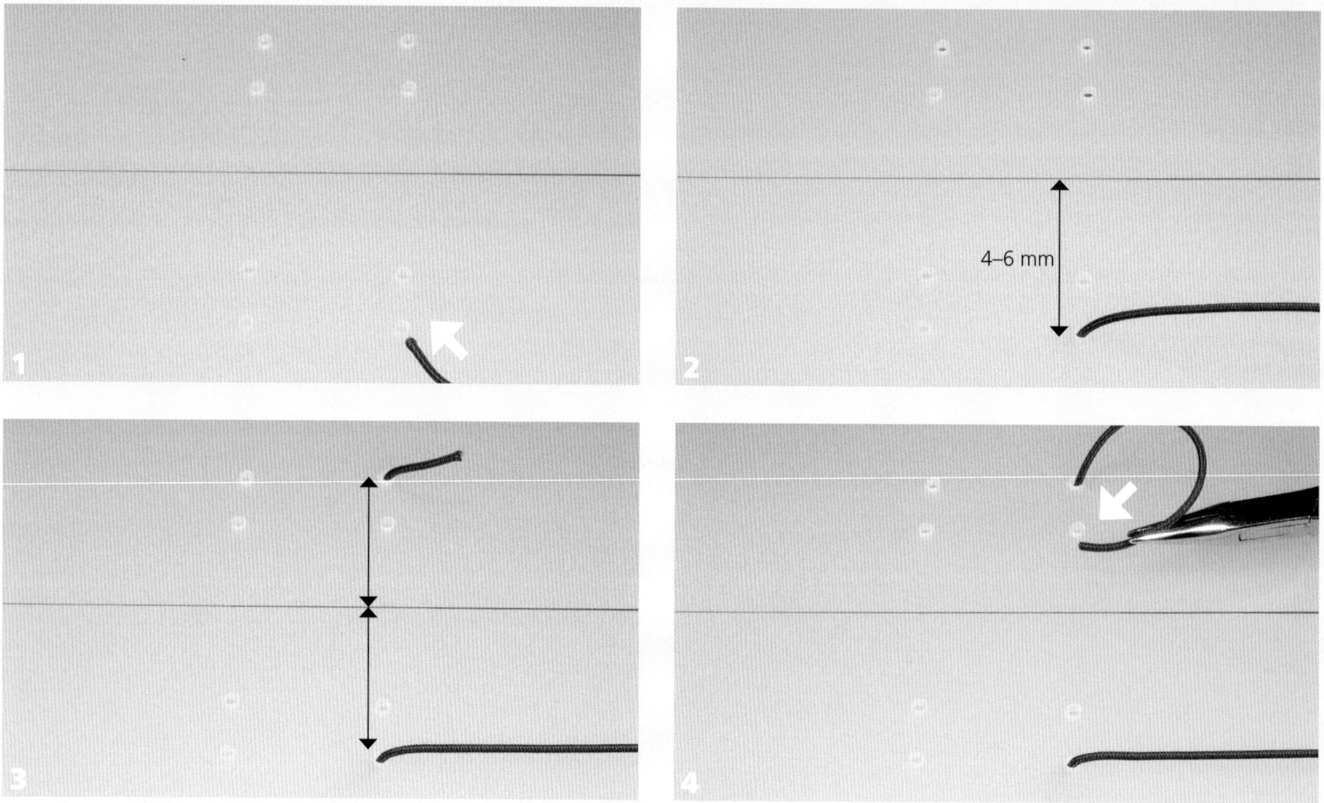

1 In a first step, the suture penetrates the mobilized flap from the outside to the inside. **2** A distance of approximately 4 to 6 mm from the incision line must be maintained at all times. **3** The second flap is pierced outward at the same distance from the incision line as the first flap. **4** The needle is turned and the second flap is pierced from the outside to the inside in a perpendicular line to the wound margin.

Schematic representation

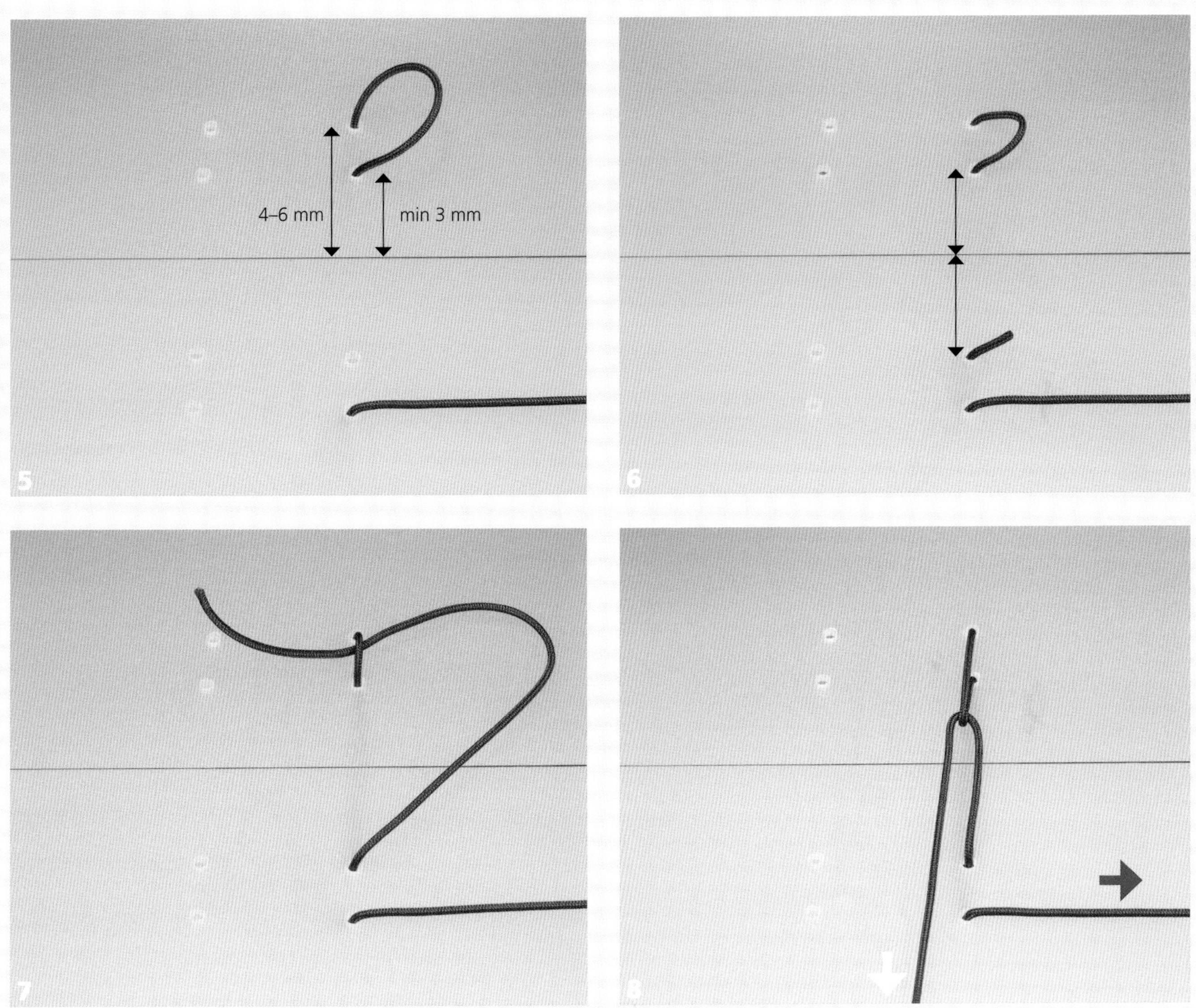

5 The distance to the wound edge should be at least 3 mm to avoid tearing the wound edges during knot formation. **6** While maintaining the same distance on both sides, the suture pierces back outwards through the mobilized flap, and the two ends of the suture are tightened until a small loop is formed on the second flap. **7** Before knotting, the thread is picked up again with the tweezers and passed through the loop of the second flap from the incision side. **8** The flaps can now be ideally positioned by pulling on both thread ends.

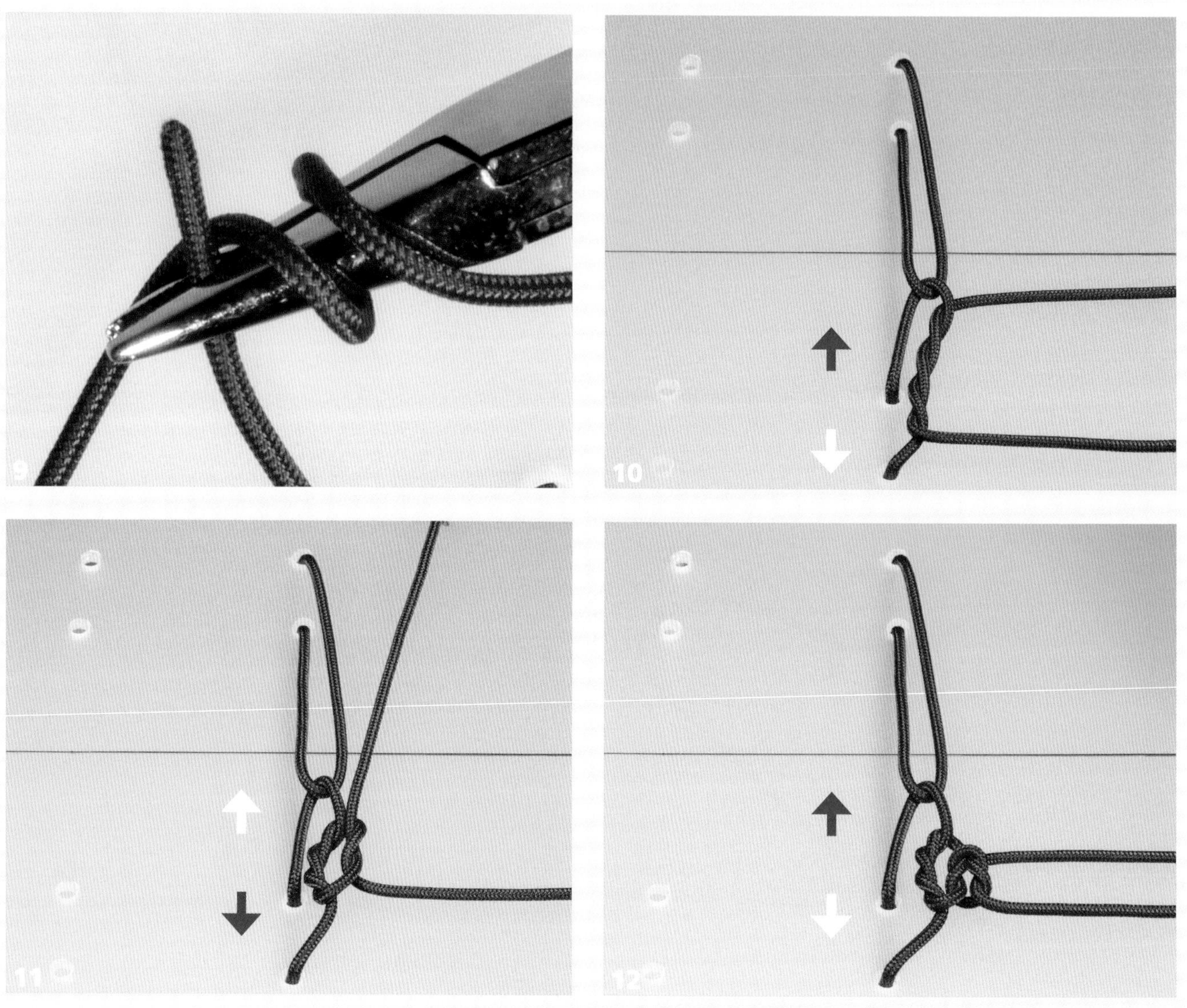

9 Finally, the knot is formed in the same way as for the single button suture. The long end is looped twice around the needle holder. The short end is grasped with the needle holder. **10** The knot is tightened and assumes a stable position. It lies straight, shows a spiral pattern, and should preferably lie on the mobilized flap lateral to the wound edge. **11** The second knot is made in the opposite direction with a throw. This ensures that it can no longer open. **12** The knot formation ends with a third safety knot in the same direction as the first.

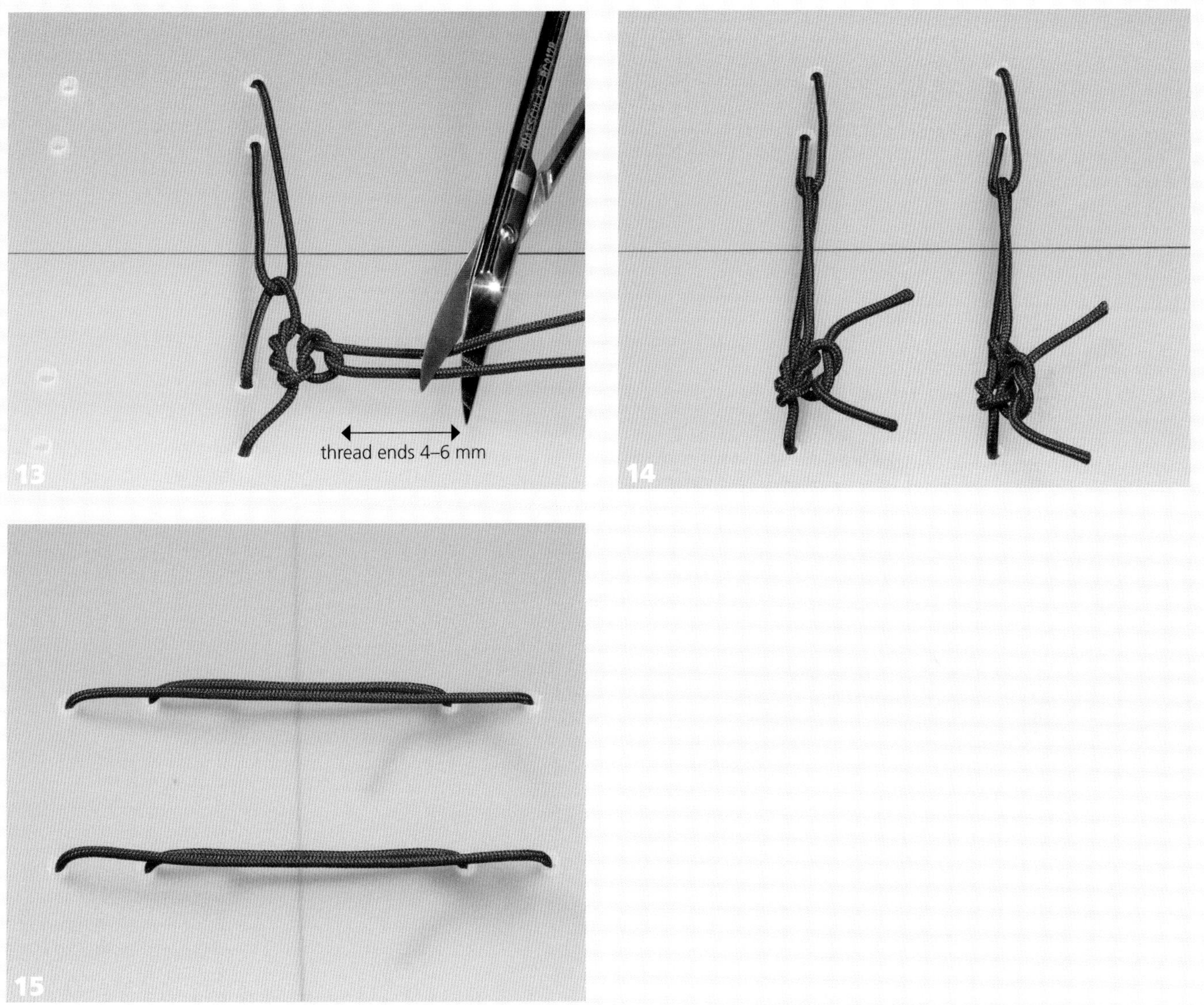

13 Finally, the thread ends are shortened with scissors to a length of 4 to 6 mm. **14** Two finished vertical Laurell sutures. **15** Two vertical Laurell sutures from "below" (tissue side).

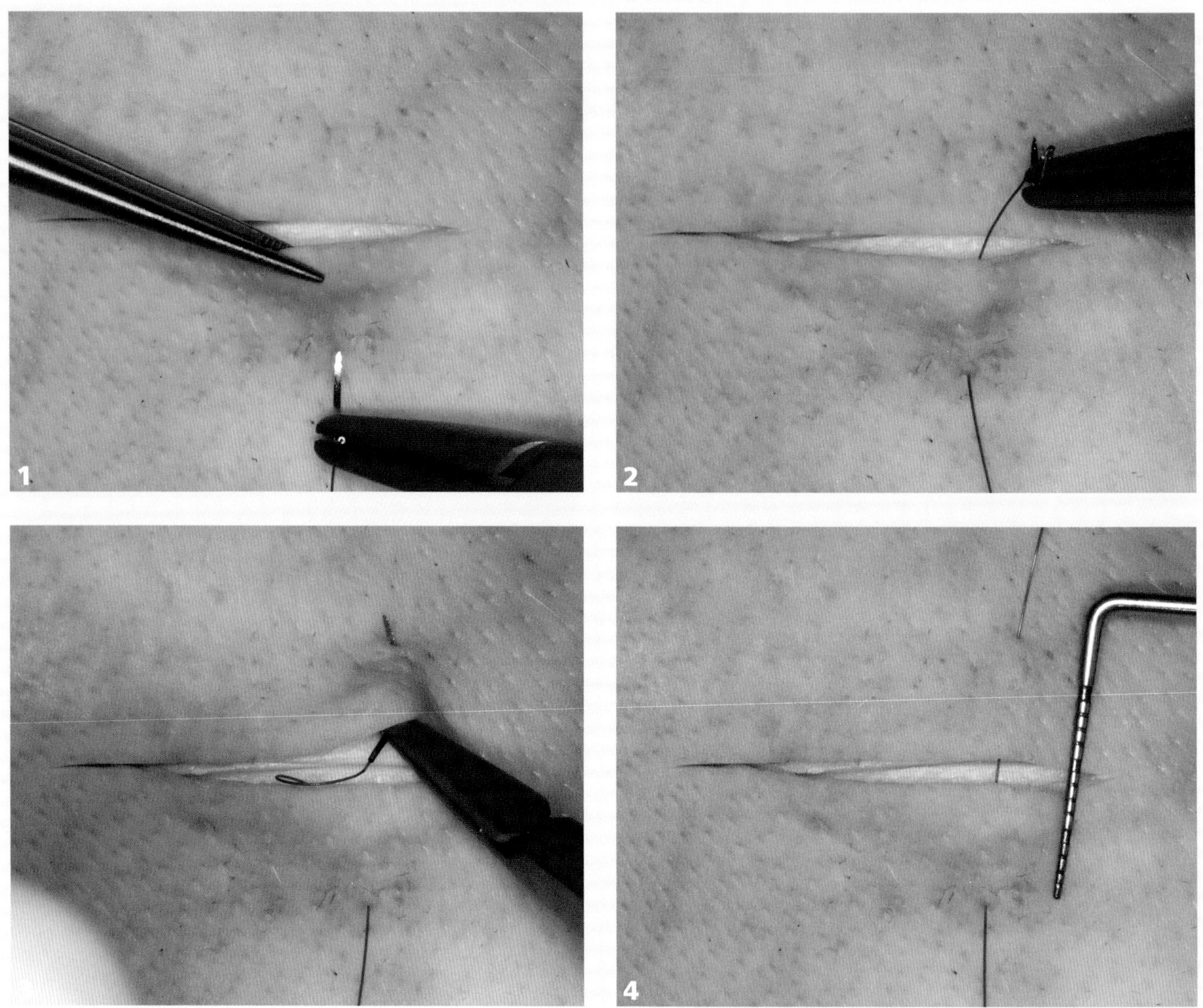

1 The first step is to pierce the mobilized flap from the outside to the inside. **2** The suture is pulled through the wound gap. **3** The second flap is penetrated from the inside to the outside at the same distance from the wound margin. **4** The distance between the incision line and the puncture site should be at least 4 to 6 mm.

Representation on the animal model

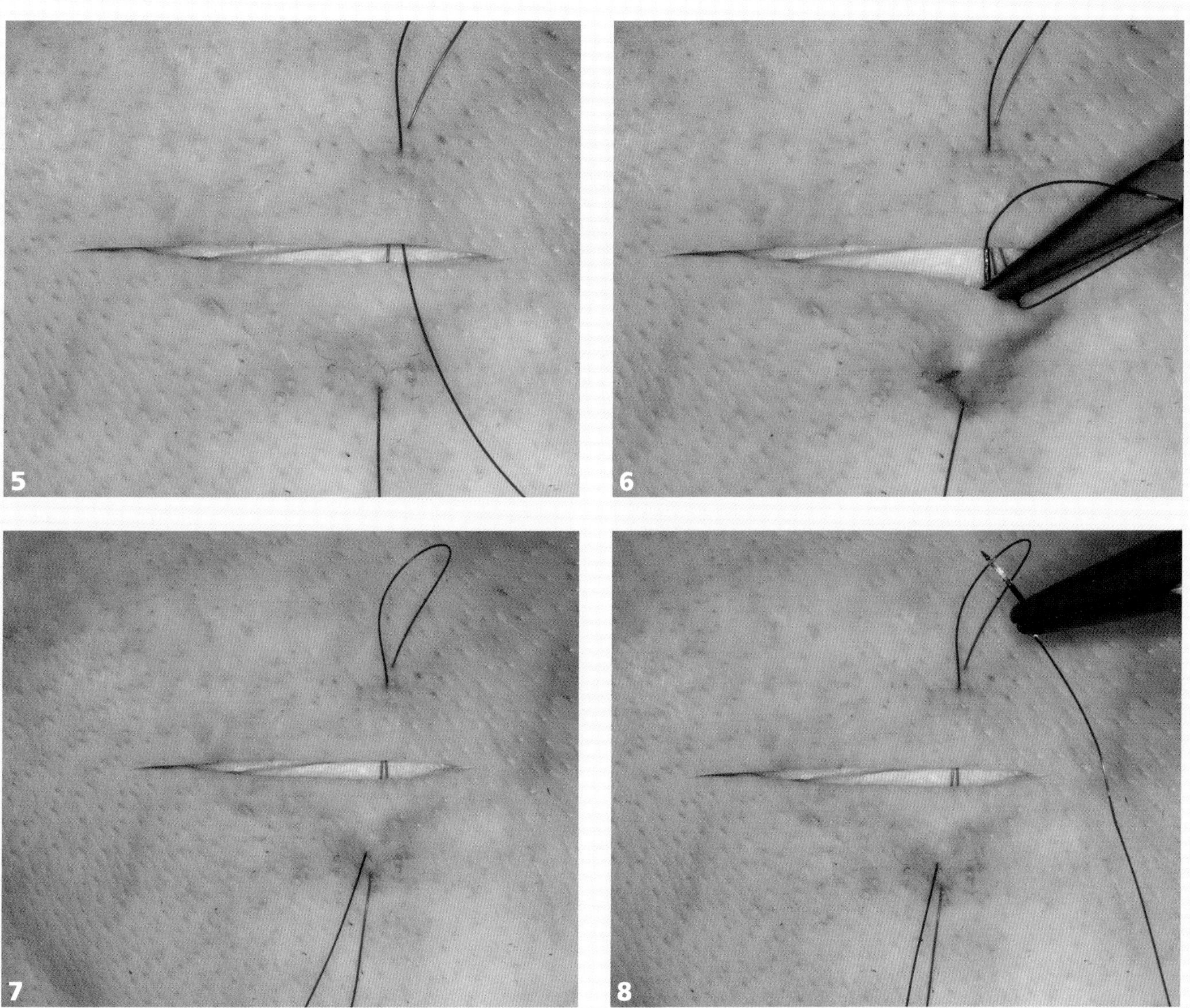

5 The suture pierces the flap again on the same side from the outside on a line perpendicular to the wound gap. The suture emerges again in the wound gap. **6** While maintaining the same distance on both sides, the suture pierces outward through the mobilized flap. **7** The distance to the wound edge should be at least 3 mm to prevent tearing of the wound edges. The thread is tightened until there is a small loop on the second flap. **8** The vertical mattress suture is followed by a single button suture. The thread is picked up again by the forceps and passed through the loop on the second flap.

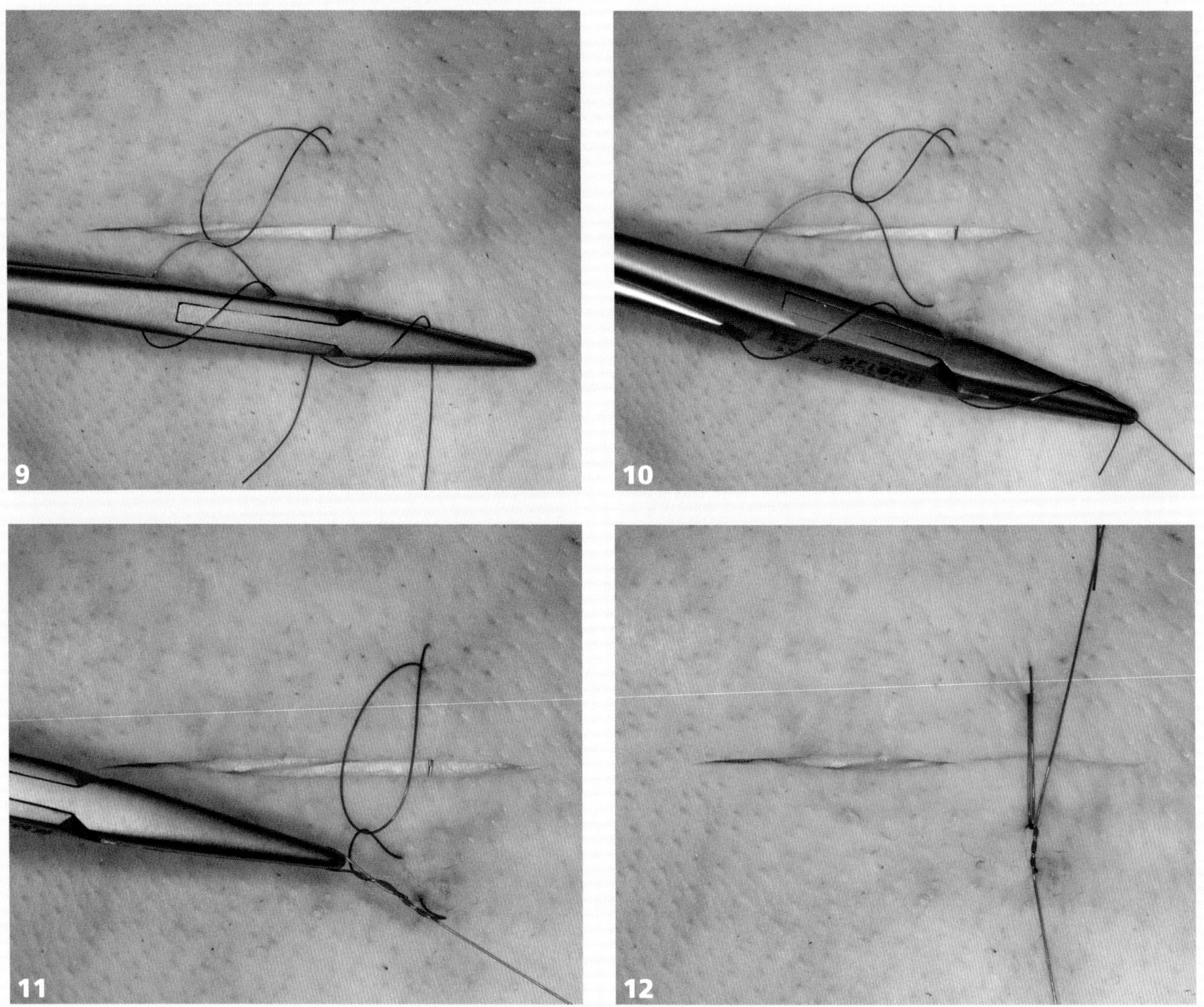

9 The knot is made in the same way as for the single button suture. The long thread end is looped twice around the needle holder. **10** The short end is grasped with the needle holder. **11** The knot is carefully tightened. **12** The knot should preferably come to rest on the mobile flap away from the wound margin and lie straight with a spiral pattern.

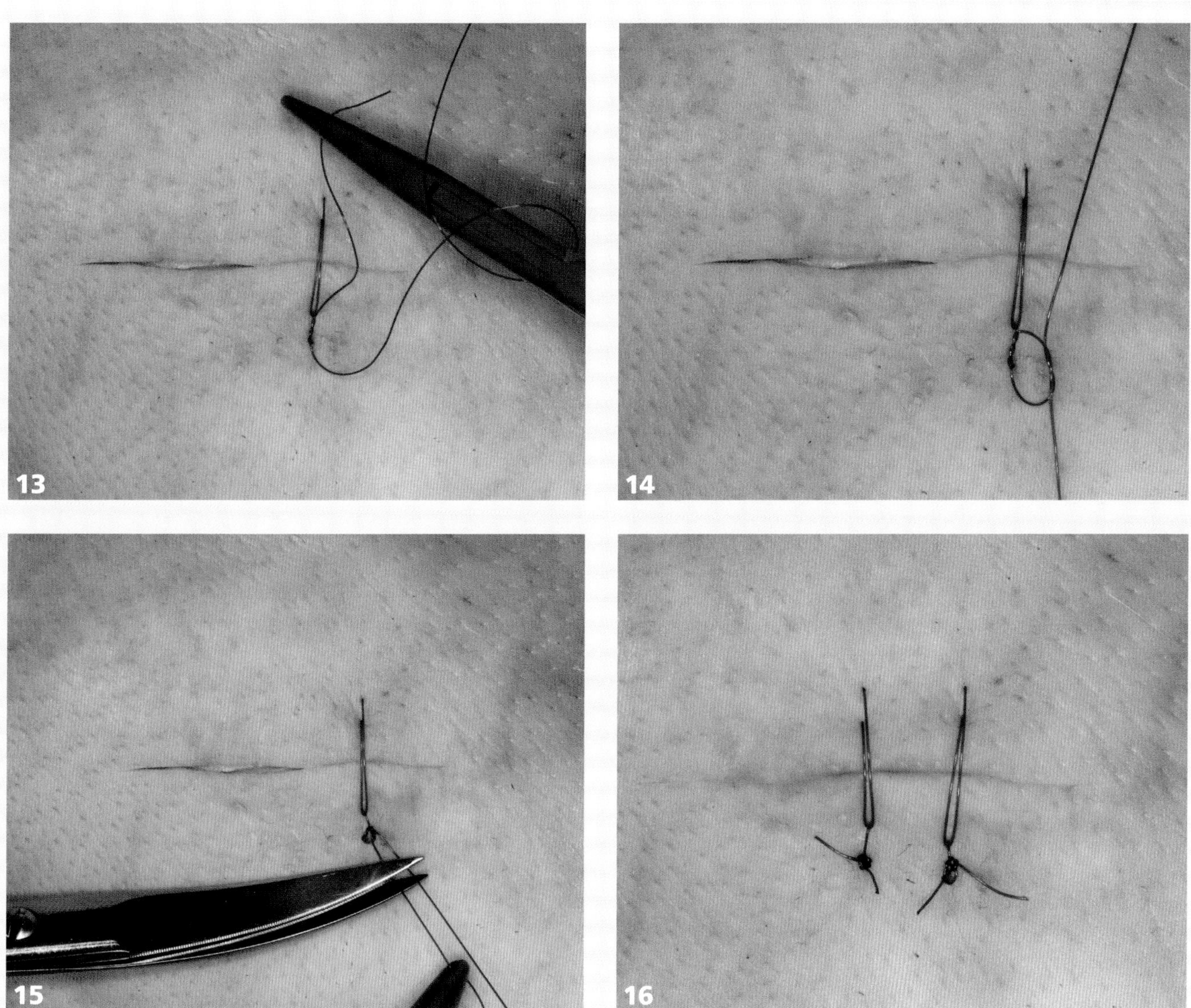

13 The second knot is made with a throw in the opposite direction to the first knot. This is now tight and can no longer come loose. **14** The third knot with a throw in the same direction as the first serves as a safety knot. This is also carefully tightened and placed away from the wound margin. **15** The ends of the sutures are trimmed with scissors to a length of 4 to 6 mm. **16** Overview of two adjacent vertical Laurell sutures.

4.4 Continuous suture | 4.4.1 Simple continuous suture*

4.4.2 Continuous interlocking suture

Indications for continuous sutures:

- Closure of long incisions that do not have great esthetic relevance
- For gaping wounds after serial extractions
- In the edentulous ridge
- For repositioning osteotomies in the maxilla

Note:

- Corresponds to a sequence of interconnected single button sutures.
- Advantage: Saves time compared to single button sutures.
- Disadvantage: If part of the thread comes loose, the tension of the thread is released in all the surrounding tissue.

White arrow: Beginning of thread
Gray arrow: End of thread

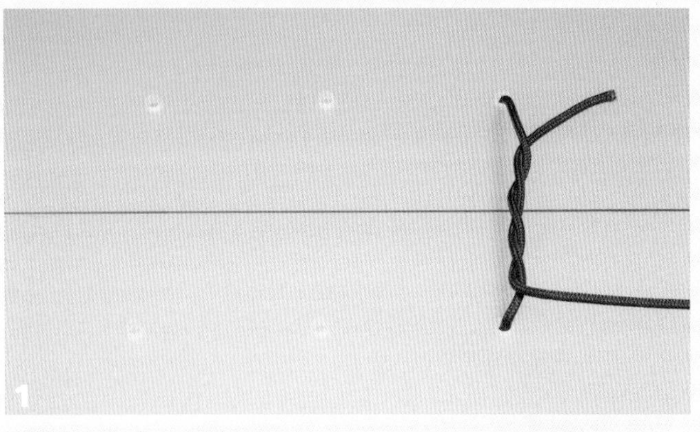

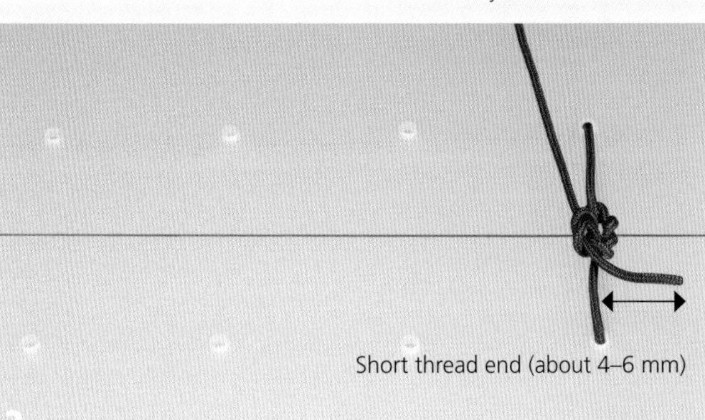

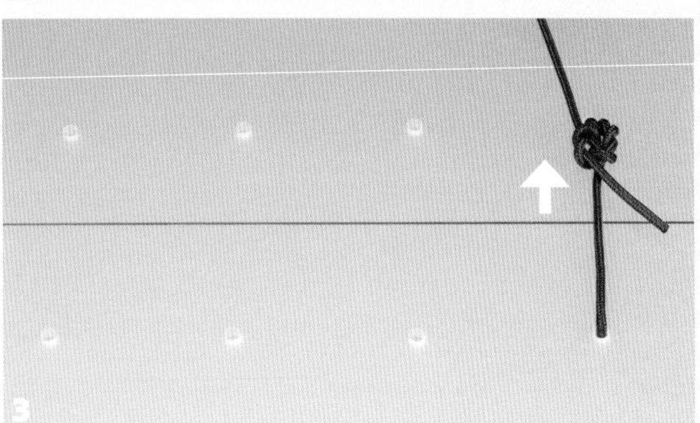

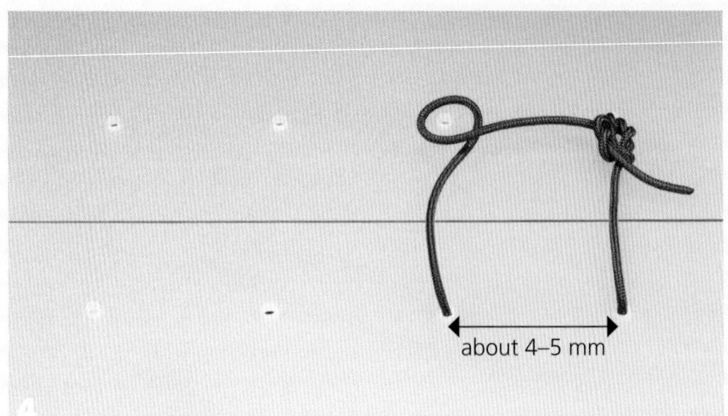

1 **The knot is made in the same way as for the single button suture. The knot is tightened and should assume a stable position. It lies straight and shows a spiral pattern.** **2** **After completing the single button suture, only the shorter thread end is cut to a length of 4 to 6 mm.** **3** **Now the knot is pulled to one side of the puncture. The knot should preferably be placed in the area of the keratinized gingiva, if present.** **4** **After a loop rotated by 180 degrees has been made as an eyelet at the level of the next puncture point parallel to the wound gap, the puncture is made on the other side of the wound gap at a distance of approximately 4 to 5 mm from the first suture.**

* Clinically low relevance compared to looped back continuous suture and therefore not shown.

Schematic representation

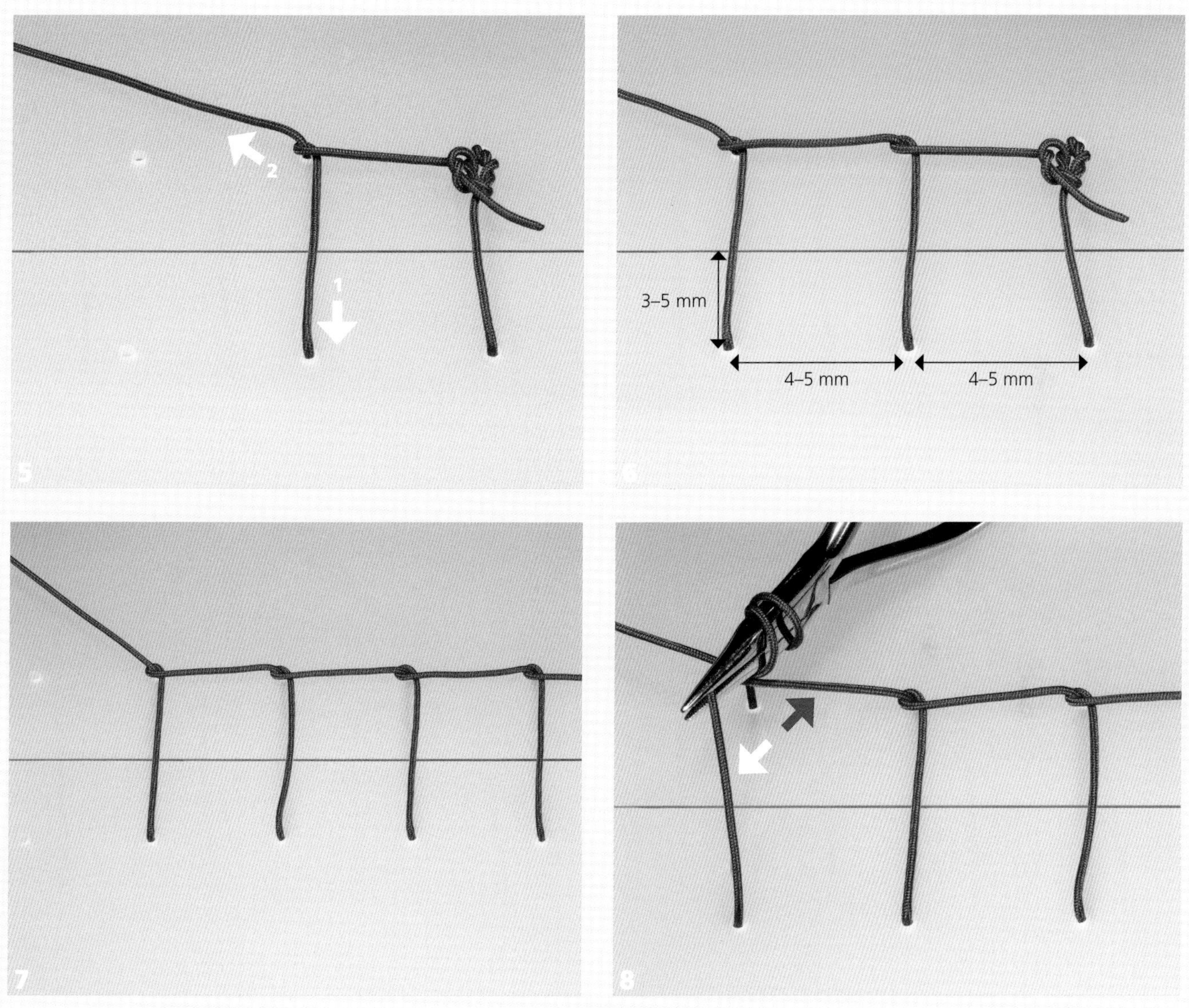

5 Now the thread catches the loop as it exits the fabric and thus fixes itself after being pulled tight through the loop turned by 180 degrees. **6** The seam is continued in this way. The consistent distance between the individual sutures, which are perpendicular to the wound edge (4 to 5 mm), is just as important as the distance between the puncture points and the wound edge (3 to 5 mm). **7** The continuous suture can be extended as desired and is limited only by the total length of the thread. **8** The continuous seam is completed with a knot in the same way as for the single button suture. The long end is looped twice around the needle holder. In this case, the short end is the last thread perpendicular to the wound edge and is grasped with the needle holder.

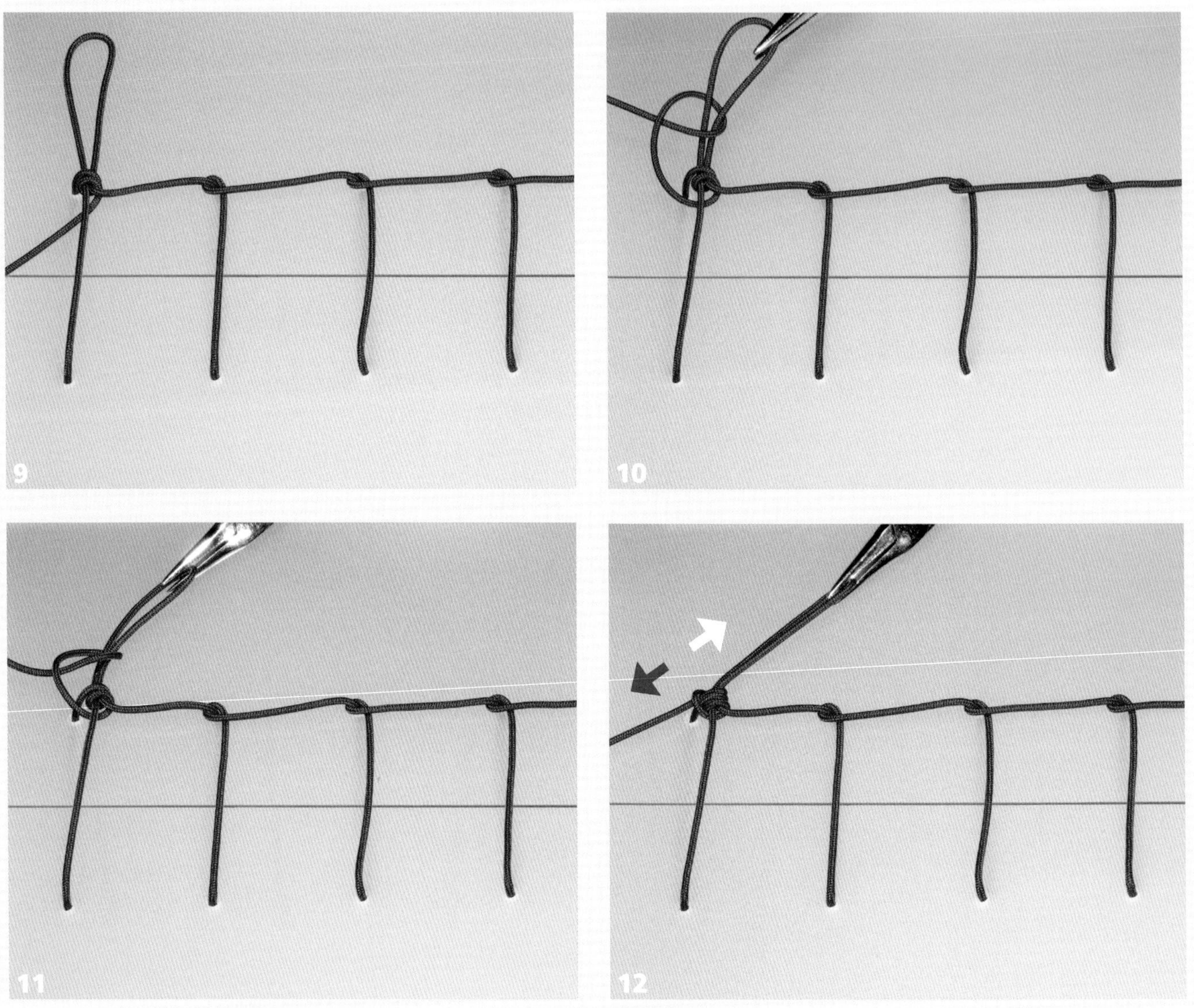

9 A loop is created, which represents the short thread end for further thread knotting. **10** Another knot is made in the opposite direction with a throw. **11** This is done in the same way as for the single button suture. **12** The second knot is firmly tightened in order not to lose the tension in the continuous suture.

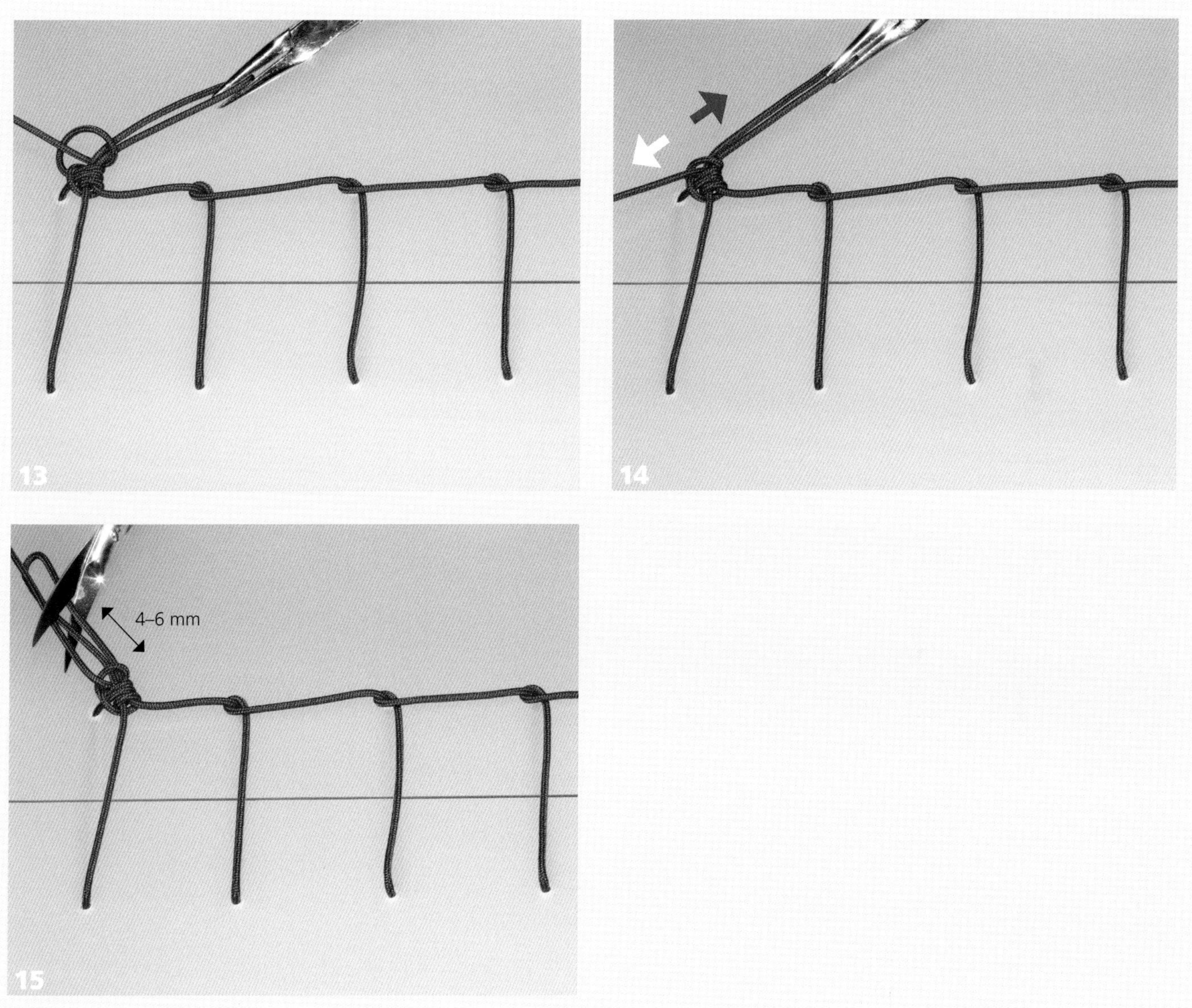

13 Another safety knot with a throw in the same direction as the first knot is performed. **14** This third knot is also tightened.
15 Using the scissors, cut the knot to a thread length of 4 to 6 mm. **Note:** Don't be surprised that the loop creates three thread ends.

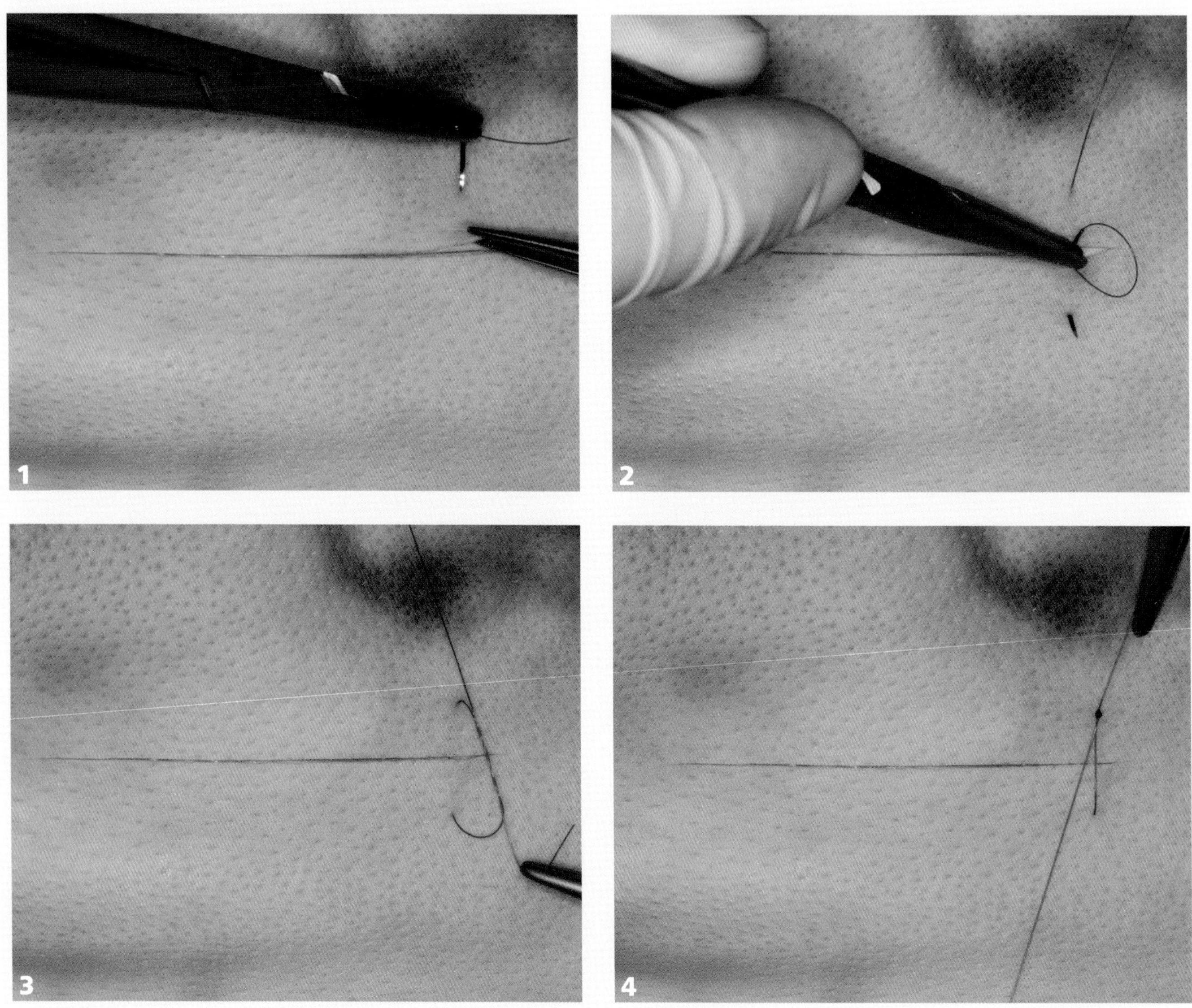

1 The flap is penetrated from the outside to the inside with sufficient distance to the wound margin. **2** The needle penetrates the second flap from the inside to the outside. The procedure corresponds to that of the single button suture. The distance to the wound margin should be the same on both flap sides. **3** After knot formation, where the long end is looped twice around the needle holder and the short thread end is picked up for pulling through, the first knot is fixed. The thread should come to rest smoothly and in a spiral pattern. **4** The knot should lie away from the wound gap (not on the wound gap). The knot should preferably be placed in the area of the keratinized gingiva, if present.

Representation on the animal model

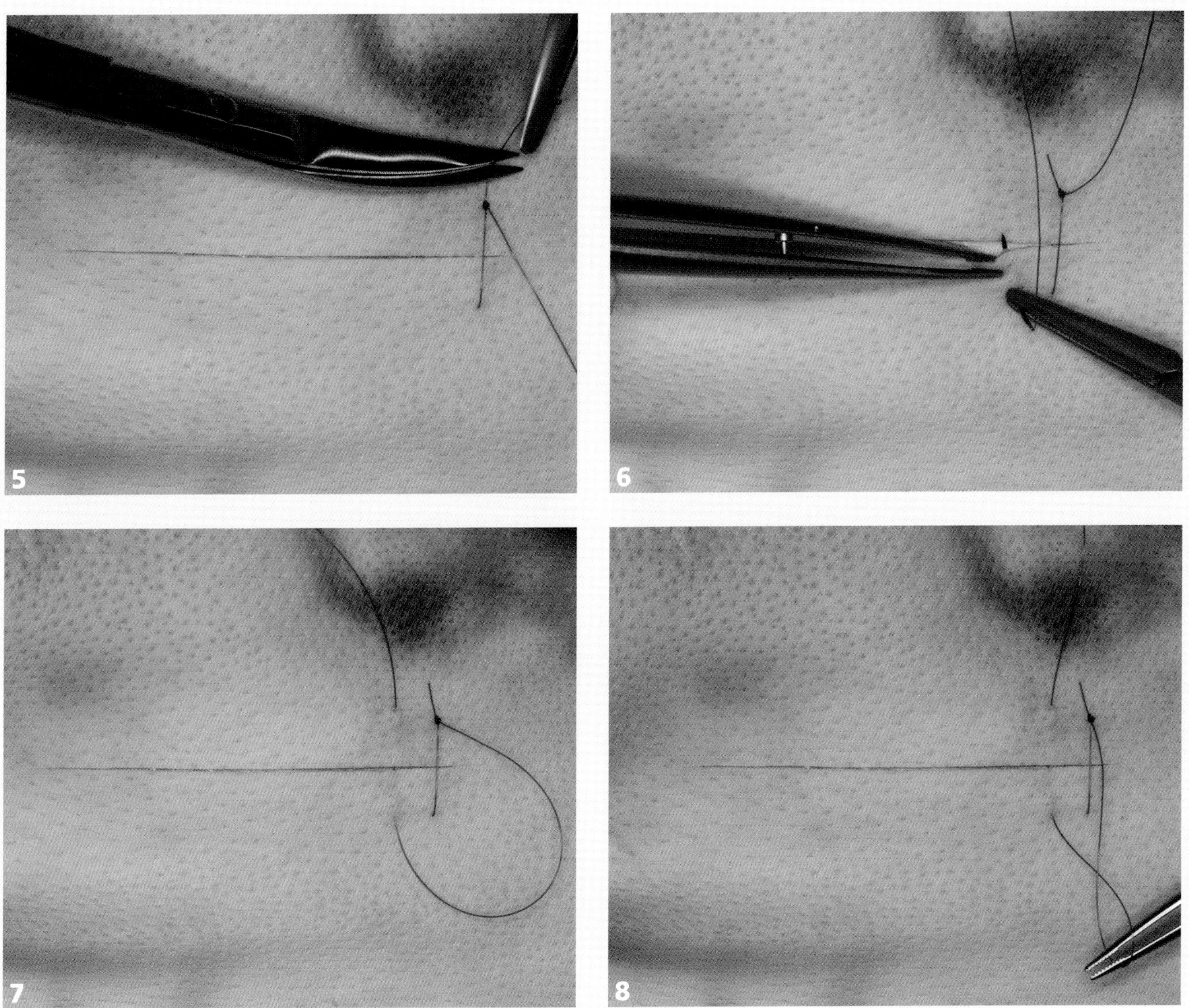

5 After completing the knot in the fashion of a single button suture, the shorter end of the thread is cut off with scissors. **6** Now, at a distance of 4 to 6 mm from the already existing suture, the tissue on the opposite side of the wound margin is penetrated with the needle from the outside to the inside at a distance of 3 to 5 mm ... **7** ... and on the other side of the wound gap, the suture is passed again from the inside to the outside. The suture is not yet pulled tight. The resulting loop has an important function. **8** After the loop has been picked up and turned 180 degrees ...

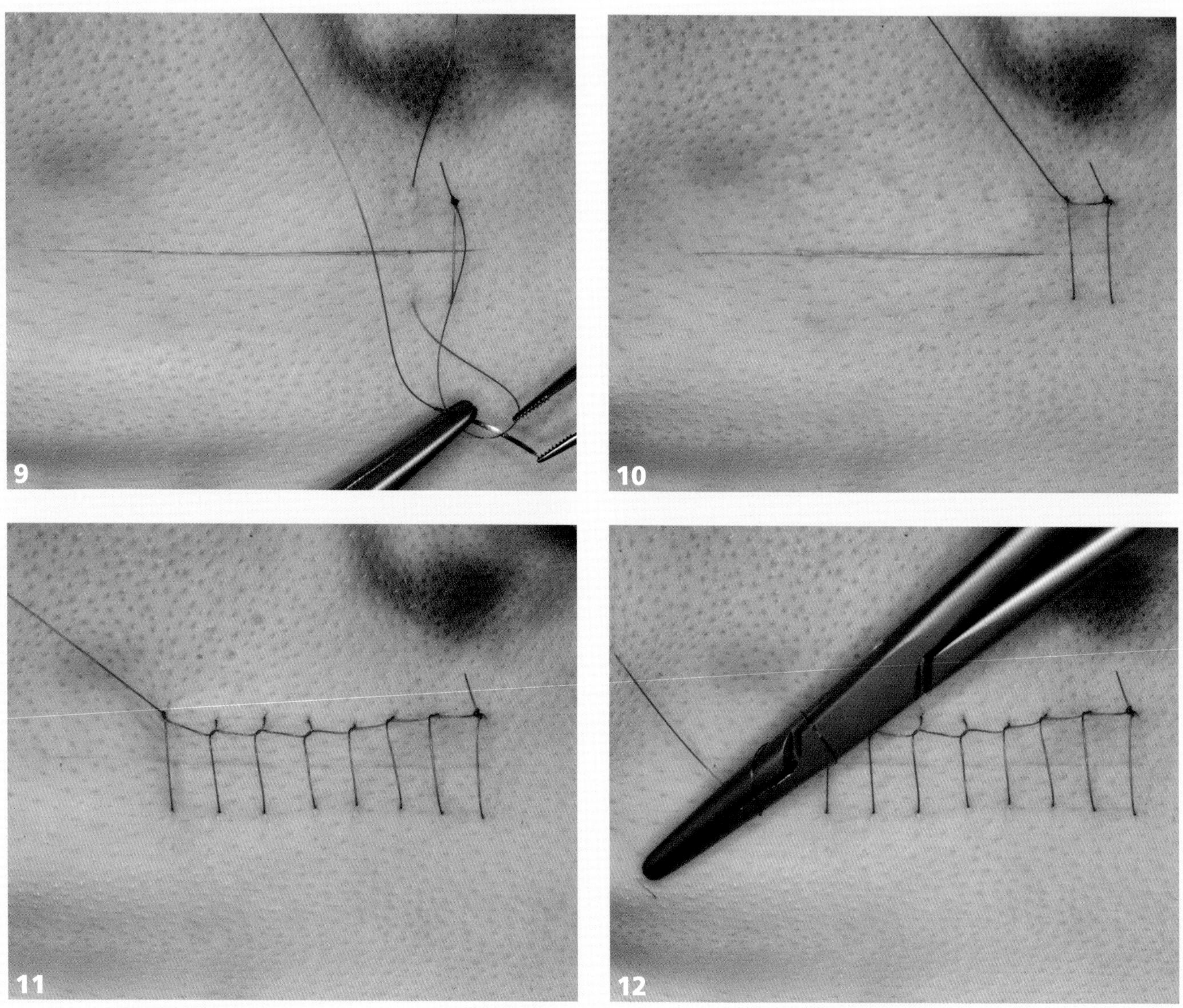

9 ... it is crossed by the thread. **10** Now the fixation can take place. Here, the visible part of the thread comes to lie parallel to the first thread. The twisted loop causes the suture to fix itself. **11** With the same procedure, the continuous suture can be extended as desired and is limited only by the thread length. **12** The end of the continuous suture is formed by a knot in the same way as for the single button suture. The long end is looped twice around the needle holder. In this case, the short end is the last thread perpendicular to the wound edge and is grasped with the needle holder and pulled through.

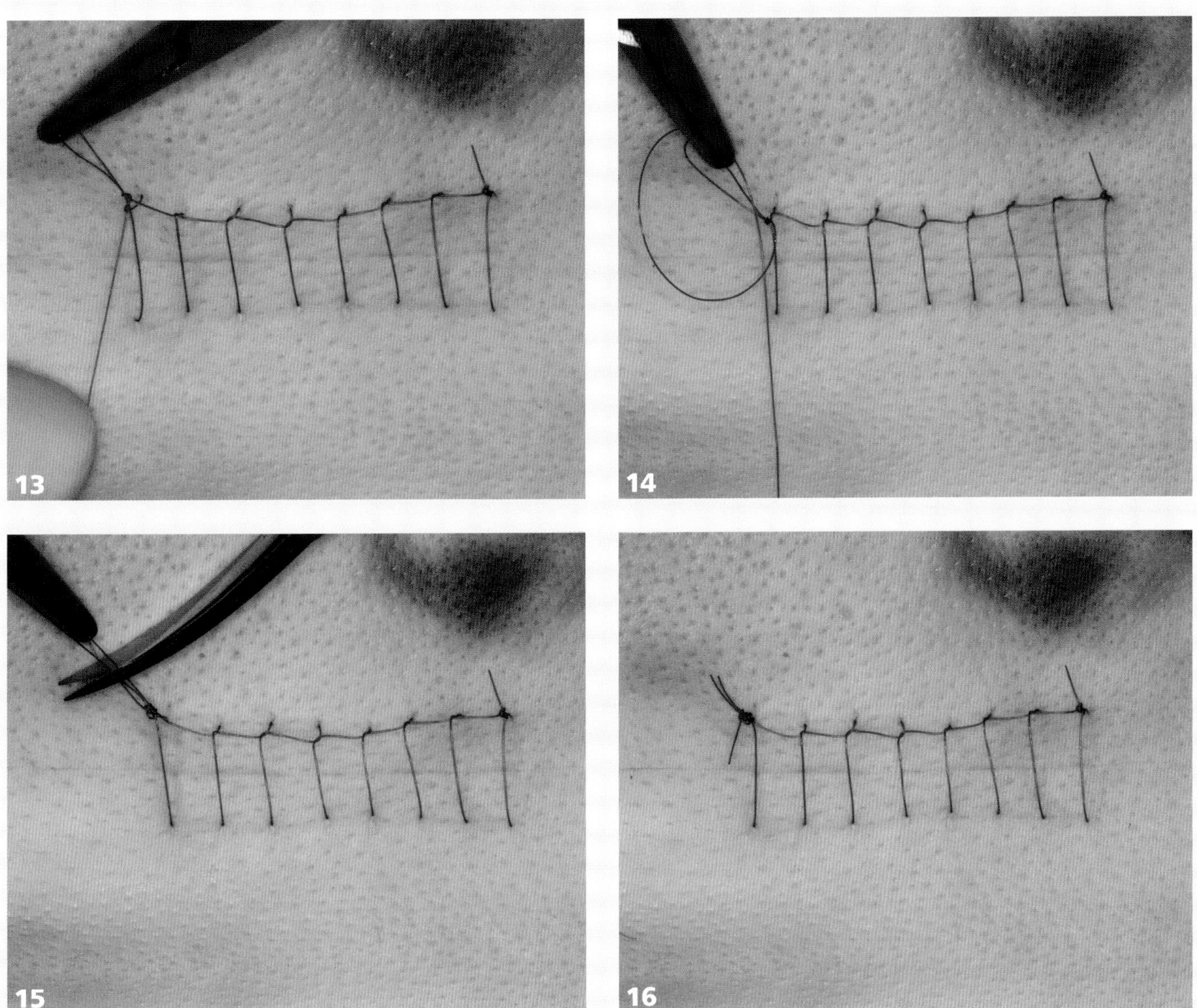

13 A loop is created, which represents the short thread end for further thread knotting. **14** The second knot is tightened firmly so as not to lose tension in the continuous suture. **15** Another knot is made in the opposite direction with a throw before the knot is cut with scissors to a thread length of 4 to 6 mm. **Note:** Don't be surprised that the loop creates three thread ends. **16** Finished continuous suture in situ.

4.5 Simple sling suture

Indications for sling sutures:

- Suitable for securing a coronally advanced flap
- Tunneling procedures
- Used in root coverage procedures
- Important for adapting the tissue margin at the CEJ
- Can be used for a single tooth or multiple teeth

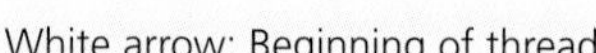

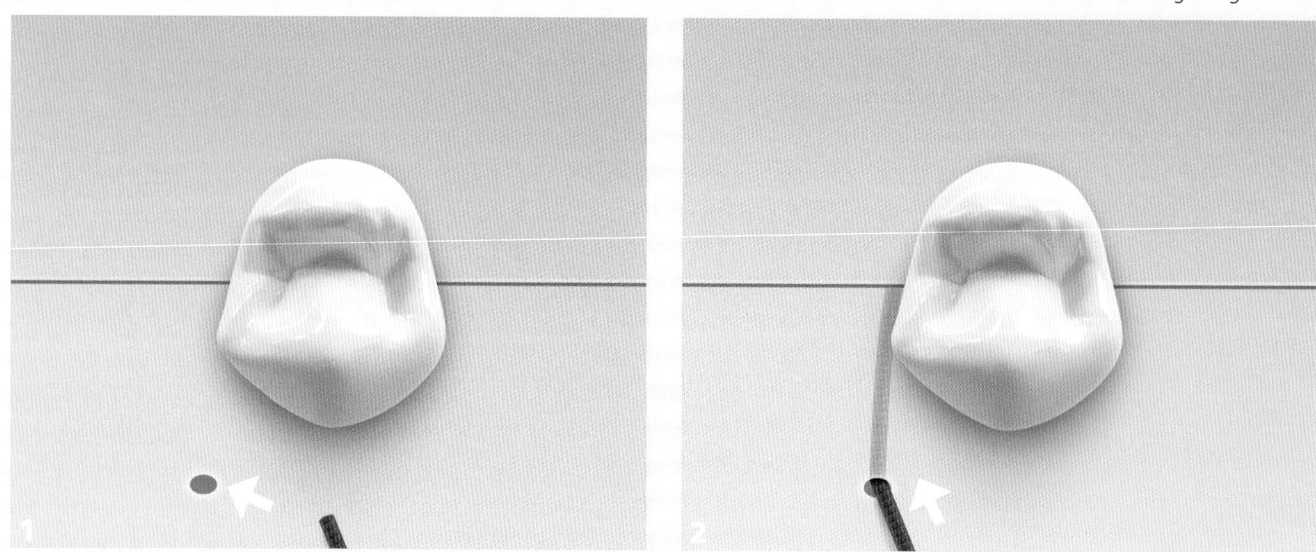

1 **The first step is to pierce the surface of the mobilized flap at the mesial or distal aspect of the tooth** **2** **The thread passes under the flap and exits at the facial flap margin.**

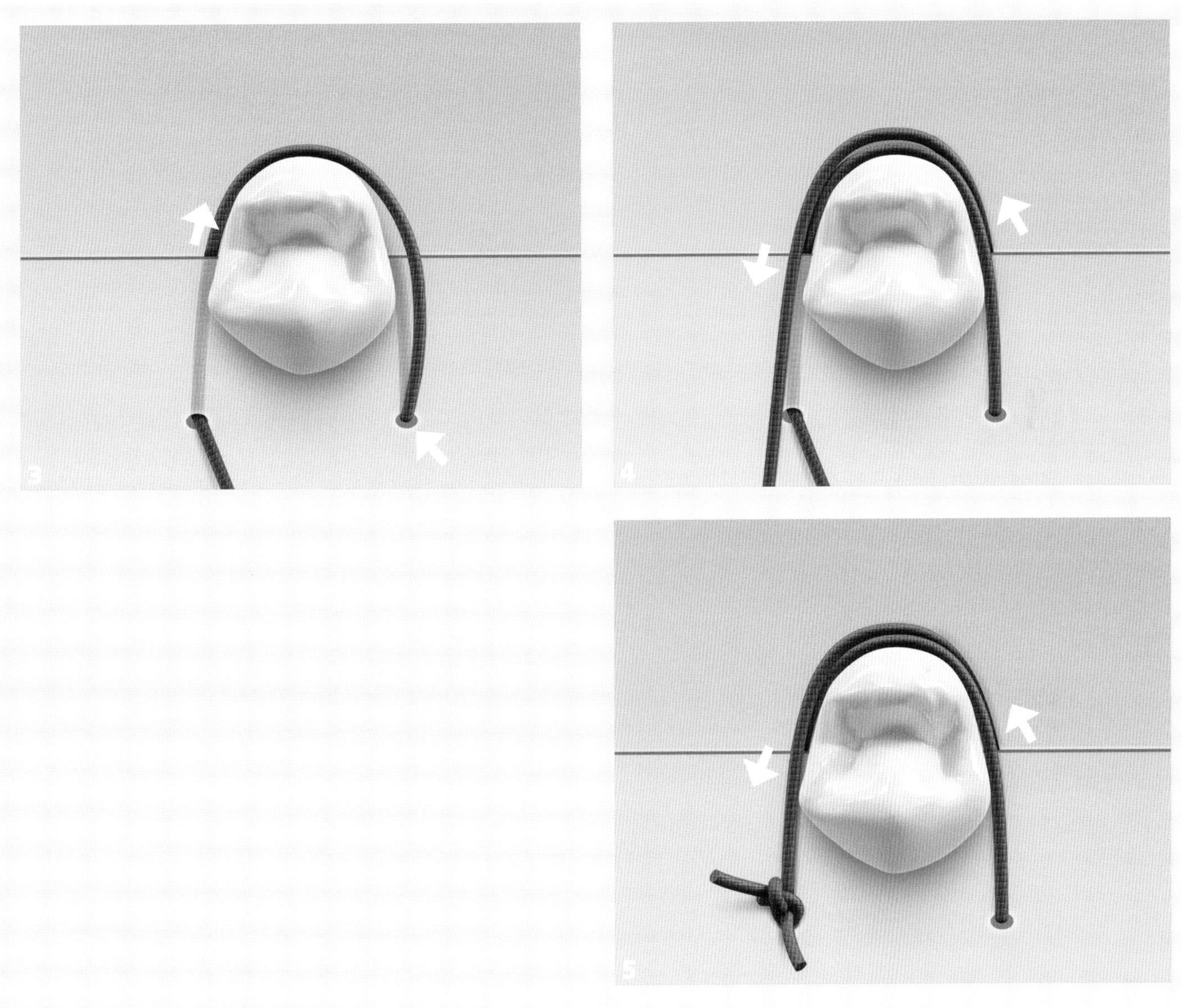

3 The suture passes around the lingual aspect of the tooth, then passes back to the facial aspect, pierces the facial surface of the flap at the opposite proximal position, passes beneath the flap, and exits at the facial flap margin. **4** The suture then passes around the lingual aspect of the tooth and back to the facial aspect. **5** After the flap is adapted at the level of the CEJ, the suture is tied.

5. Time to Suture: The Most Important Facts in Brief

- KISS: Keep It Simple, Stupid. The simplest and most uncomplicated suitable suture is the best (Ethicon: Surgical Knot technique).
- After tying, the suture should lie securely; it should not slip, and the knot should not come loose.
- The ends of the sutures should not be cut too short. Suture ends that are too short disturb the soft tissue, causing irritation that often leads to ulcer formation. On the other hand, longer suture ends make it much easier to take up the sutures during removal, and they can be shortened at any time.
- Use suture material that is as thin as reasonable for the task at hand.
- Always use a magnifying aid when placing delicate structures (eg, loupes with a light system or a surgical microscope).
- Try to suture in the attached gingiva, as this is where the visible scarring is least.
- When suturing, pierce the tissue at least 3 to 5 mm from the wound edge.
- Use your thread as effectively as possible to avoid major waste.
- Use monofilament, non-absorbable sutures whenever possible.
- Always use high-quality, securely closing, and sharp surgical instruments to ensure well-defined margins. Any closure is only as good as the suture material allows.
- Do not use the suture as a rope to close the wound (the exception is stitching around vessels to stop bleeding). The thread and its sutures are there to keep the flap ends tension-free in as immobile a position as possible.
- To prevent the first knot from reopening while the second one is being prepared, it is recommended to use the 2-1-1 method* when tying a surgical knot up to and including 5/0 thread thickness and according to the 3-2-1 or the 3-1-2 method for 6/0 thread thickness and thinner.
- Additional knots beyond those mentioned in the previous point do not improve the holding power of a knot but only increase its thickness. This can be useful for mattress sutures to make it easier to find the thread again.
- Monofilament sutures can be left in situ for longer because—unlike multifilament sutures—there is no reaction with the surrounding tissue. As a general rule to avoid wound reopening, the sutures should never be removed too early.
- Always allow sufficient time for wound closure during the procedure.

* The numbers indicate the number of times each knot is thrown over, with the first and third knots tied in the same direction and the second knot tied in the opposite direction.

6. Complication Management

This chapter is dedicated to techniques for avoiding and overcoming any problems that may arise during suturing. Basically, tension-free wound closure is the key factor for success. This can sometimes be time-consuming and complex, particularly in the case of augmentation measures. However, time is well invested to avoid wound dehiscence. In all cases of dehiscence, close monitoring by the practitioner is necessary.

Possible causes of wound dehiscence

- Postoperative bleeding and hematoma formation in the wound area after surgical intervention
- Mechanical injury to the wound and lack of immobilization (eg, due to sharp edges or cleaning of the surgical area by the patient)
- Wound infections
- Insufficient and poorly fixed sutures, wrong suture material, wrong suture technique
- Incorrectly fitted restoration or appliance, such as a temporary denture or splint

---

6.1 Thread breaks during suturing

A thread breaking during suturing can have various causes. It may be that the thread was too thin, and therefore could not withstand the loads. In this case, a thread with the next greater level of thickness must be selected.

If the suture tears, in most cases it is because too much traction was used when attempting to close the wound. The practitioner is inclined to compensate for the lack of flap mobility by pulling the suture tightly. However, this is absolutely the wrong way to close a wound adequately and permanently. Initially, the primary wound closure may appear good. After several hours, or at most over the next few days, the tissue yields to the traction, and the sutures slowly glide through the soft tissue. Consequently, wound dehiscence occurs, which often leads to failure of the surgical procedure. In these cases, work must be done on the soft tissue rather than on the suture. This starts with meticulously planned incision placement and adequate dissection and ends with tension-free wound closure with the correct suture material. If tension-free wound closure cannot be achieved, the wound area should be reopened and the dissection extended until tension-free wound closure is fully guaranteed.

6.2 Wound edges open in the Initial healing period

If, contrary to expectations, the wound area opens, a distinction must be made as to whether only a marginal aspect of the wound is open and the wound edges therefore do not gape completely or if the wound edges protrude completely and the underlying surgical area is exposed.

6.2.1 Wound edges are only superficially exposed

An attempt can be made to re-adapt the marginally protruding wound edges using additional suturing. Primarily mattress sutures and single button sutures are used for this purpose. Of course, care must be taken to avoid creating too much tension on the wound edges again; otherwise, the problem is very likely to recur or worsen. In some cases, it might be better not to disturb the site.

6.2.2 Wound edges protrude and partially or completely expose the surgical site

Based on the type and location of the procedure, the next steps depend on the contamination of the exposed tissue. In the case of major augmentation procedures, an attempt can be made to remove superficial tissue and to disinfect the exposed tissue with targeted measures (eg, with povidone-iodine or chlorhexidine), in order to subsequently apply a tension-free wound closure. In any case, antibiotic therapy should support the surgical measures. To avoid further mechanical damage, the patient should perform a gentle rinse with saline or chlorhexidine for 60 seconds. In addition, Solcoseryl can be carefully applied several times a day with a cotton swab. Solcoseryl is a paste containing a dialysate from calf blood to promote healing and polidocanol 400 for rapid-onset and sustained pain relief. After application, patients should not drink or eat anything for about 2 hours so that the medication can take effect.

These measures are an attempt to close the wound again. A successful, durable wound closure cannot be guaranteed in this way. Nevertheless, it is worth a try. Alternatively, inserted material (eg, bone substitute material, an implant) must be removed and the wound subsequently reclosed. After appropriate soft tissue healing, the procedure can be performed again.

6.3 Wound edges open after suture removal

If a wound opens after several weeks, long after suture removal, a late infection can usually be assumed. In addition, an area of augmentation with sharp edges can cause initially healed wounds to open. The dehiscence that occurs should be treated.

6.3.1 Infection

If an infection is involved, irrigation of the wound area with povidone-iodine and saline is recommended following an incision some distance from the area of augmentation. A drain should be inserted to ensure drainage. After 1 to 2 days, the drainage is cleared with renewed irrigation with saline. If the drainage of the saline is no longer cloudy in color and clear liquid is discharged, drainage can be discontinued. If this is not the case, the drainage should be renewed until this condition is reached. After removal of the drain, the incision site will close on its own within days. Accompanying antibiotic therapy with a broad-spectrum antibiotic is strongly recommended.

6.3.2 Opening due to sharp edges/pressure points

The treatment of choice for exposed hard tissue grafts is to debride the bone until bleeding occurs. In addition, the sharp edges that have led to dehiscence must be rounded and smoothed. After disinfection, an attempt can be made to close the wound again. Accompanying broad-spectrum antibiotic therapy is strongly recommended.

As a basic principle, care must be taken to ensure that provisional restorations, splints, and similar devices only rest passively and do not exert any pressure on the tissue in the wound area.

If wound closure is no longer possible, it is recommended that the patient should perform a gentle rinse with saline or chlorhexidine for 60 seconds. This is always an attempt to preserve the graft as best as possible. The success of these measures, however, cannot be guaranteed. Alternatively, graft removal may become necessary.